Table of Contents

Part I: A Developmental Look at Signing with Your Child — 1

Each chapter gives an overview of your baby's physical and linguistic development and abilities for the age. Specific signs, activities, and strategies appropriate for each age are discussed.

Chapter One: What Is Baby Sign Language? — 3

This chapter includes an overview of baby sign language—the history and research behind it, and what parents need to know.

Chapter Two: Birth to Three Months—I'm Just Not Ready Yet, But... — 29

This chapter describes the development of your very young baby and why you should be talking to your baby as a preparation for signing with her.

Chapter Three: Four to Seven Months—I'm Ready to Start — 45

This chapter gives you the basic steps to start signing with your baby and includes tips to create a basis for lifelong communication.

Chapter Four: Eight to Twelve Months—Watch Me Sign — 81

This chapter explains your baby's development between eight and twelve months and why your baby is now ready to sign back. It also helps you to understand how to use your baby's communication clues to increase your ability to understand her.

Your baby is primed for communication and is motivated by all the new things she is learning. This chapter explains why your baby is exploding with abilities and why signing comes more quickly at this time. It gives you specific strategies to help develop these abilities to help you both communicate better for life.

Your baby is ready for speaking. You may wonder how to transition from signing to talking and how signing can benefit your baby even once she can speak. This chapter covers these issues and also provides you with activities to increase your baby's ability to learn to speak.

Your toddler is speaking and interacting with new things every day. He still may sign things for a long time. But as he continues to grow in his communication abilities, things will change, and he will master speech. This chapter explains the things you and your child can do to use his signing abilities to facilitate future learning.

This chapter discusses the issues specific to children with special needs and what resources parents have to help them sign with these wonderful children. Signing can be an amazing experience for children who otherwise would not be able to express themselves due to physical or mental limits.

Part II: Baby Sign Language Dictionary 199

The dictionary includes a complete list of all the signs displayed in the book, along with many more that you will find useful in your signing experience. The dictionary is divided by activity, so that all the signs you might use for a specific activity are included. This means that some signs that are appropriate for multiple situations are repeated in the dictionary.

Acknowledgments

No one writes a book alone. You sit in front of the computer with your thoughts and type, but that is just one part of the process. I'd like to thank all the people who influenced and helped me on this journey.

Thanks to the pioneers in signing with babies. Thanks to Dr. Joseph Garcia and his generous and loving soul. Without his first thoughts about using ASL for signing with babies, my relationship with my children would be less fulfilling. Thanks to all the parents I have interacted with over the past several years as I taught them about signing with their babies and shared with them the *Sign Babies ASL Flash Cards*. Your love and commitment to your children are inspirational.

Thanks to those who have worked directly with the book. Thanks to Bethany Brown for having vision and faith as my editor, and to Peter Lynch for finding me and taking the project to the press. Thanks to the following brave souls who read the book in its draft form and were kind enough to give feedback and encouragement. Thanks to Kim Fries, CCC-SLP of Little Hands . . . Make Big Words for your expertise in ASL and speech development. Your help on the Special Needs chapter was indispensable. Thanks to Kimberly Fakler for your input on Special Needs as well. Thanks to Barbara Grannoff of Sign-A-Lot for your expertise in ASL and for your encouragement. Thanks to Dr. Anne Ure for your expertise in early childhood development. Thanks to Tricia Taylor, Sheia Korth, Todd and Daisy Stonely, Shannon Eden, Melanie Fergason, and Stephanie Lowe for your experience as parents who sign with your children. Thanks to Dr. Kari Lawrence and to Dr. D. Todd Whiting for your medical expertise. You helped me give birth and take care of all of my babies–including this book. It has been a wonderful experience working with all of you. Thanks to Lori Sume, my illustrator and friend. Lori's art makes *Sign Babies* possible.

Finally, thanks to all those at home who made it possible for me to write:

My husband and my children have given me the inspiration and the space to write. My mother and my in-laws have been there to support me with care for my family. And, thanks to God for the opportunities that have made it possible for me to learn and sign with my own babies. My life with them would be less rich without baby sign language.

Preface

For thousands of years, parents have struggled to communicate with their babies and have searched for ways to connect with them. Mainly this was done through parents doing all the talking and the figuring out and babies doing all the listening. But recently, in an amazing breakthrough, parents are realizing that communicating with their baby is not just a one-way interaction.

Babies have always been trying to let their parents know what they are thinking. Some parents have made their lives easier by understanding what certain grunts, looks, sounds, and gestures of their baby might mean. This one-way communication was better than nothing and it gave parents a chance of understanding what one cry meant over another.

However, the secrets of how to create two-way conversations with your baby at an earlier age are being opened now, with an innovative approach to communicating with babies. Parents are learning that if they use basic signs with their baby—also called baby sign language—they can begin the conversation much earlier, as much as a year earlier. This book describes a progressive understanding of what children do naturally and details how we can use these natural tendencies to create two-way conversations by introducing specific, simple signs that allow parents and children to communicate.

The national news media has featured this innovative concept of baby-parent communication on every major morning news show, as well as on the evening news. Celebrities appearing on Jay Leno and David Letterman shows have talked about how their babies were able to communicate at nine and ten months using these methods.

The interest in baby sign language is certainly growing because many parents are able to communicate with their babies much sooner. But you might be asking, "What's all the fuss about? Is this something that I really want to do with my baby? Can I really communicate effectively with a baby younger than two years old by using my hands?" Maybe you have been enticed by the buzz and want to know what baby sign language is all about and what you can expect from your baby.

This book is a great place to start answering these questions and it is also a great resource for age-specific guidance. Because there is a great difference between a four-month-old and a twelve-month-old, this book is specifically designed to explain your baby's developmental stage and to tell you what you might expect from your efforts to communicate with your baby. It explains the methods and strategies best suited for your baby's development and provides you with signs and activities to use with your baby at her specific age.

The Foreigner in Your House—Your Baby

If you think of your baby as a visitor from another country, it is easy to see what it is like for her. She has taken a plane trip to your home—maybe even a very bumpy ride—and is now thrust into a language and culture that she has never encountered before. She has to learn the language, the customs, and the traditions to function well in your home.

Now, how do most people react when they meet someone who can't speak their language? The clichés are that people tend to speak louder, speak directly at the person, speak slower, and use their hands to make themselves understood. Actually, some of this is effective. You will learn in this book how to use your hands, speak directly at your baby, and speak slower so that your baby can learn quicker (no need to be louder). Your baby will also learn to use her hands, look at you directly, and slow down in order to be understood. Soon, you will have the ability to communicate with each other before your baby can speak.

My own experience

It has been more than a decade since I first heard about signing with babies and started doing research and collecting information on the subject. In the ensuing years, even more has been written about baby sign language. In particular, a breakthrough book had been widely distributed: *SIGN with your BABY* by Dr. Joseph Garcia. This book changed my life and the life of my son. It was the first book to use American Sign Language (ASL) as the basis for communicating with hearing babies and it was also the first book to explain not just why parents would want to do so, but how to do it. (ASL is the most commonly used language for Deaf Americans and Deaf Canadians.)

Based on what I learned in the book, I began using basic ASL signs with my son when he was just seven months old, creating a way for us to communicate. When my son was born, the doctor took one good look at him and said, "This baby has an attitude." She was right. He was born with an insatiable need to be understood. For the first six to eight months of his life, his father and I had played a guessing game trying to understand his needs. And, at around nine months, when he could finally communicate with us using signs, it felt like a gift from the heavens and turned my experience of being a parent from a nightmare to a dream.

Friends of mine began to ask me how things had turned around and I started teaching them about the joys of signing with babies. I became a certified baby sign language instructor and taught hundreds of families how to have the same bliss in their lives. At the same time, my son and I were growing in our experience of learning about each other and about the world.

We have an extensive library of books and we often incorporated signing into our reading sessions (more on how to do this in later chapters). But I did encounter one difficulty. The books often included concepts or objects or animals that I did not know how to sign. I knew thousands of signs but had never had the need to know whether there was a sign for armadillo until we read *Goodnight Gorilla*. It was also hard to find books that included the signs that we were working on most.

With these issues in mind, I created a book for my son by taking a simple 4 x 6 photo album and placing pictures of things we were signing in the book, along with the word for that item. As a writer, I have published several books and articles on various subjects, but this little book I created for my son turned out to be the most important book I ever created. A friend of mine saw it and said, "I want one! When you get it in the stores, I will be your first customer."

The original photo album morphed into the *Sign Babies ASL Flash Cards*. These flash cards are based on two ideas: keep things simple so parents can understand what they need to know—even at 3:00 a.m.—and make sure that babies who can't read can still use them.

Until then, no materials had been designed specifically for signers who could not read. You had to be literate in order to learn to sign from books or other available materials. Babies and young children can't read, but they *can* learn to sign if they interact with their parents who are signing and have tools adapted for their abilities.

The experience of signing with my son and creating the *Sign Babies ASL Flash Cards* helped me focus on my 3:00 a.m. age-appropriate philosophy. Everything that *Sign Babies* creates should be understandable at 3:00 a.m. and should be age-appropriate. There are wonderful dictionaries of thousands of ASL signs available, but most of the signs are not ones parents and children find useful and they are written in a specific language unique to ASL (which most parents don't understand because they are not students of ASL). There are even some good books on activities to use to sign with your baby, but the activities are age-specific.

With the help of our first Sign Babies Flash Cards, my son learned to sign more than forty signs, including things such as **MILK**, **EAT**, **APPLE**, **BANANA**, **SLEEP**, **MOON**, **STARS**, **PLAY**, **CAT**, **DOG**, **PLEASE**, **THANK YOU**, and so forth. When he turned sixteen months, he began to speak all the words he knew how to sign—more than one hundred words! Additionally, he decided to learn the alphabet and numbers one through nine on his own. By eighteen months, he could say more than two hundred words and started putting multiple-word sentences together. He mixed words and signs to express himself. His first four-word sentence was "Drink go fall down" when his sippy cup fell off the high chair. Because he could sign and talk early, we had lots of fun together and many fewer tantrums.

Parents' Biggest Question and Why This Book Works So Well

Over the past five years of teaching hundreds of parents to sign with their babies, I have spent a lot of time answering the same types of question: "My baby is six months; what should we sign?" "My baby is fourteen months; is it too late, and what should we start with?" A baby at six months is very different from a baby at fourteen months, and each parent needs specific information about what and how to sign at that age and about what to expect from the experience.

This book provides the answer to all of those questions. Because you might be starting to sign at birth, or you might be starting at twelve months, you need information that is pertinent to you and your baby right now. This book gives you the information you need to know for the stage your baby is in today. You will understand not only what to sign, but why it works and how signing integrates into your baby's overall development.

How to Use This Book

The goal of this book is to break things down by age-appropriate categories so that you know what to do with your baby today. It includes basic information on the how to's of baby sign language and then gives you specific activities you can do with your baby at each age.

Part I gives you a developmental look at how to sign with your child. Each chapter provides an overview of what is going on with your baby developmentally during a specific age, then describes the basics of signing at that age. There is also a chapter dedicated to children with special needs, because, depending on their physical or mental limitations, you might need to modify your signing strategies. Finally, each chapter includes specific signs for use during activities such as mealtime, bath time, playtime and so forth, and explains why these signs and activities work well at this age. Baby sign language is not rocket science, but knowing a few good tricks and tips makes it easier. Remember, keep things simple and follow the easy-to-accomplish steps for the greatest success.

Part II includes a baby sign language dictionary of all the signs displayed in the book, along with many more that you will find useful in your signing experience. The dictionary is divided by activity so that all the signs you might use for a specific activity are included. This means that some signs that are appropriate for multiple situations are repeated in the dictionary. No need to search.

This book is designed so that you can read it from cover to cover to get a complete feeling for what works to facilitate communicating with your baby. Or, if you are swamped with life and need to just get down to what you need to know right now, you can flip to the chapter that corresponds to your baby's age and dig in (if you need information from previous chapters, it is noted at the beginning of each chapter). When you get a chance, go back and read the other chapters for additional information and tips about signing.

Note: When you see words that are bolded and in capital letters (**APPLE** or **MORE**, for example) these are the words that you will sign with your baby. Sometimes, you will sign only one word in a sentence that you speak to your child. As your child becomes more accustomed to signing, you will sign more than one word per sentence.

Enjoy the Journey

Thank you for picking up this book. My hope is that you enjoy the journey that you and your child are on. Parenting is an amazing experience and signing with your child can really enhance the trip for both of you. This book will help you understand ways to enhance your experience and gain more joy and insight. Peace to you and your family.

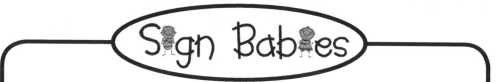

Part *I*

A Developmental Look at Signing with Your Child

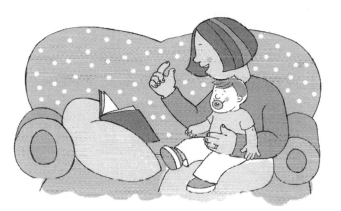

This section provides a developmental look at how to sign with your child. Each chapter includes the following for the specific age:

☆ Overview of what is going on with your baby developmentally
☆ Steps for signing
☆ Tips for success
☆ Specific signs to use during certain activities
☆ Explanation of why these signs and activities work well at this age

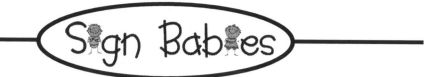

Chapter One

What Is Baby Sign Language?

Over the past few years, baby sign language has been featured everywhere from the news to big-screen motion pictures. All these sound bites and clips probably intrigued you, but they did not give you a great idea of what baby sign language is. You may be wondering whether there is a "language" called baby sign language or whether it is based on another language. Or, you may be worried that if you sign with your child, he might not talk. Some people even worry that if they sign with their baby, their child will go deaf.

This chapter takes a look at what baby sign language is, its origin, why it works, and what myths might be out there about it. It explains what it can do for you and for your baby, as well as what it won't do. In short, it gives you the information that you need to decide whether signing with your baby is right for you. Let's get started.

What Is Baby Sign Language?

Before we discuss what baby sign language is, let's clarify what the terms *language* and *speech* mean. We all use language to understand what is said to us (*receptive language*) and to express ourselves (*expressive language*). *Language* is how we communicate with others using words, signs, or writing. Language includes the types of words we use—nouns, verbs, adjectives, adverbs, how many words we use, how we put the words together to form thoughts, and so on. *Speech* is how we pronounce words and show the language we have acquired. Interestingly, we have some language before we have speech, meaning that before we can speak, we can communicate with others by using gestures, grunts, and visual cues. This is the predicament that babies are in—they have things (language) to express, but very few ways to express them.

Baby sign language is a way to communicate with your baby before he can speak. It uses your baby's natural abilities and tendencies to increase the clarity of your daily interactions. Babies naturally try to communicate their wants and needs. As a part of their attempt to communicate, they naturally use their hands. Who hasn't seen a baby raise his arms to show that he wants to be picked up? What mom hasn't had her child emphatically gesture to grab something that he wants but which is out of reach?

Baby sign language taps into these natural tendencies by empowering your baby to communicate needs, wants, and even complex thoughts with his hands. It bridges the gap between the time when your baby can't communicate with words and the time when he can be clearly understood.

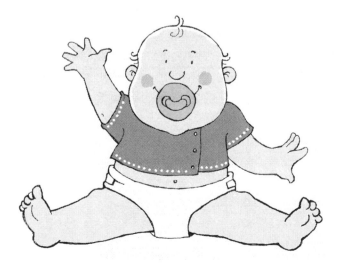

Think about how empowering this can be for your baby. Instead of crying and hoping you can guess that he needs his diaper changed or wants to have some applesauce, he can tell you. As a parent, in many cases, you will no longer have to guess what your baby wants. He can tell you. You don't have to be standing in the grocery store line with a screaming baby wondering whether he is hungry or tired or bored. He can let you know.

If you choose, baby sign language can be the beginning of a wonderful experience learning a new language—American Sign Language. Or if you only want to use it as a bridge during the time when your baby cannot communicate with words, it works wonders. In either case, baby sign language is fun and easy for both parents and children to learn and do. It takes a lot of the guesswork out of being a parent because it has the power to stop tantrums and start conversations.

In addition to enhancing communication, baby sign language may have additional benefits for you and your child. We will discuss these later in this chapter. However, the best benefit is a closer bond with your child.

AHA!

American Sign Language is the third-most used language in the United States, after English and Spanish. It is also used in Canada. More than one million Americans use ASL. So your baby has a head start on his language requirements in high school and he might make some great friends in the Deaf community along the way.

Tapping into Your Baby's Natural Abilities Using Simple Signs

In order for anything to work for parents and babies, it needs to be simple and natural. You're in luck. Signing is something that comes naturally to babies. They point at things they want, wave with their hands to say "bye," and clap to show excitement. These are all signs—it is that simple. You are only taking advantage of their in-born tendencies by teaching them simple signs for things they want. It takes a little patience and dedication on mom and dad's part, but any baby can do it. And it fits right into your daily routine. You don't "make time for sign." You just add signs to the conversations and communications you already have with your baby.

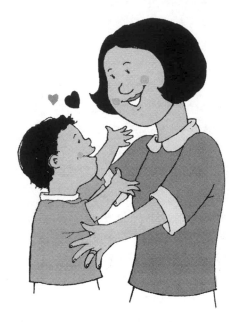

A lot of parents worry that using baby sign language means that they will have to spend a lot of time learning another language. That's not true. The signs you will use are borrowed from American Sign Language (ASL), a beautiful and rich language. However, you will not generally be using the syntax, structure, or other linguistic qualities of ASL. You are borrowing only a few signs from a vast language. After signing with your baby, you may decide to go on and learn more about ASL and Deaf culture. I recommend it. But if you just want to understand what your baby's needs are, that is a wonderful reason to sign with your baby.

Remember, *this is not rocket science*. It just takes a few simple steps and some tips to make it work. I have broken the process down into age-specific guidelines so that you can know what works best at what age.

Benefits of Signing with Your Hearing Baby

A few years ago, I stood before a room of successful businessmen to discuss my *Sign Babies ASL Flash Cards* and my business needs. These were men who had started banks, software companies, and other businesses and who had seen fads come and go. The first question I was asked was, "How many deaf babies are born in our town?" The men thought that my product was intended for deaf babies. I smiled and said that I did not know but that it did not matter. Eyebrows went up around the table. Then I explained that *Sign Babies* was focused on teaching hearing parents of hearing babies how to sign with their children to facilitate communication before babies can speak. I went on to explain the benefits of signing with hearing babies. By the time I left, every man at the table was sold on the concept. Here is what I told them.

Hearing babies who sign with their parents and other caregivers have a unique opportunity to learn to communicate their needs and wants and thoughts long before the average hearing child can. Besides the ability to communicate, there are these added benefits.

AHA!

There is a difference between the words *deaf* and *Deaf*. The capitalized form refers to deaf persons belonging to the community—also known as Deaf culture—who use ASL as the preferred means of communication. The lowercase form refers to those who have partially or completely lost their sense of hearing. A person can be deaf and not consider himself Deaf if he does not belong to the Deaf culture and does not use ASL to communicate.

Babies who sign

☆ Speak at the normal time or sooner than their counterparts who do not sign.

☆ Have larger vocabularies when they do begin to speak.

☆ Have more interest in reading.

☆ Have better skills in spelling and reading.

☆ Score higher than their nonsigning counterparts on verbal and language tests and have higher IQ scores even as old as age eight (see Table 1).

☆ Have a better sense of self-confidence because they can get their needs met.

☆ Have parents who are less frustrated, because they spend less time in the guessing game trying to figure out what their baby needs.

☆ Have a start on a second language, which develops more of the brain earlier and promotes lifelong language learning abilities.

☆ Develop both sides of their brains at a higher rate (recent brain scans show that babies who sign have increased activity on both sides, which may occur because signing is visual, motor, and linguistic in nature).

☆ Those who live in bilingual households have an easier time transitioning between the languages when the same signs are used with both languages.

☆ Have a close bond with their parents because they can spend more time communicating with each other.

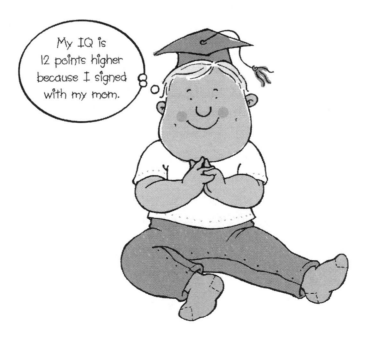

TABLE 1:
Verbal Abilities of Children Who Don't Sign versus Children Who Do Sign

Age	Developmental Norm[i]	Signing Children
12 months	Possible 2–3 spoken words	25 signs/16 spoken words[ii]
18 months	6–15 spoken words	79 signs/105 spoken words with some sentence development using both words and signs[iii]
24 months	50 spoken words/2–3 word sentences with a vocabulary of 150–300 words	Speech like 27–28 month old[iv] (200–300words[v]) (3–5 word sentences with a vocabulary 200-500 words)
36 months	Understands 800 words/ Uses 3–5 word sentences easily	Speech like 47 month old[vi] (up to 1500 words[vii]) (almost total control of everyday language)
8 years	IQ Score of 102 for control group	IQ Score of 114 for signing group[viii]

The Zero to Three website is a great resource to help you know what your baby should be doing during the first three years of his life. Please visit www.zerotothree.org/. Additional research and information on the results of signing with hearing babies is also located in Appendix C.

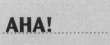

AHA!

Each child learns differently. Some learn by reading or seeing, some learn by listening, and others learn by doing. Baby sign language uses all three modalities: hearing language (we say the words), seeing language (we sign the words), and doing language (the child signs the words) to maximize the exposure and learning of language.

Signing has short-term benefits for your baby—the reduction in frustration and the ability to communicate—that are really important. It also has long-term benefits—increased vocabulary, IQ, and interest in reading—that will help your child as he grows and matures. What you are doing now will help lay an important foundation for your child's educational mindset. He will enjoy learning and will develop the necessary skills to learn well.

In addition to the benefits for your child, signing with your baby will help you have a more enjoyable relationship with your child. You will be less stressed out and will be able to understand his specific needs instead of guessing what that cry at 3:00 a.m. means. As your baby grows, you will have less of the "terrible twos" to deal with than other parents. This is because most of the tantrums come from your baby's inability to specifically tell you what he needs. Without this skill, he is left with what he knows—crying. If you teach him to sign, he will have another tool to use to let you know what he needs and that means fewer tantrums.

A final thing to consider is that even if you are already in tune with your baby, using baby sign language allows your baby to communicate his needs to others who don't have your sixth sense for your baby's needs, but who have learned a few

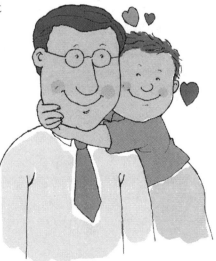

basic signs (some signs are so intuitive that even a person who does not know sign can guess what the sign means). That is very important for making your baby independent.

When Will Your Baby Begin to Speak?

Speaking is one of the last skills your baby will master because it is one of the most complex skills to learn. He must learn to master his tongue, cheeks, lips, and breathing, while directing airflow to make a noise. Speaking is a very complex dance of muscle control, so it is no wonder that it takes such a long time to master. But, in contrast, one of the first things your baby learns to do is to gain control over his hands. His hand movements can become coordinated enough to make a basic sign somewhere between four and eight months and to make more complex signs somewhere between seven and twelve months. That is much sooner than when your baby will be able to master all the body parts required for speaking. Although he is learning all the movements that are required for speaking, he is still acquiring the ability to communicate and is learning the language game. He is learning how to get what he needs and how to respond to his own thoughts. This will help him to speak better and have a larger vocabulary when his body catches up to his thoughts.

Longitudinal research funded by the National Institutes of Health studied signing children for an extended period of time. The children who signed spoke sooner than their counterparts who did not sign. The additional benefit was that during the time they could not speak, the signing children could communicate. When they began to speak, they had larger vocabularies, learned new words faster, and spoke in more complex sentences (see Table 1).

There are good reasons why your baby will speak sooner if you sign. Think about this: When you sign with your baby, you are not being silent. You are speaking directly to him. He can see your mouth, hear your voice, and see the sign. He is actually getting more linguistic input than most babies receive. Often I see parents talking to their kids with their backs turned, while they are on the phone, or while the child is distracted. None of these are optimal situations for learning to speak. On the contrary, when you sign with your baby, you will be looking at him, and he will be looking at you. You won't be distracted by something else and he will be concentrating on your face and hands. He will see and hear you speaking, which will help him learn to communicate.

Additionally, you are engaging your baby in a conversation at a much earlier age. Because you expect him to respond at some point, you are inviting him into the conversation. You are also empowering him to select the topic of conversation at a much earlier age. Once he begins signing, he can initiate and direct your conversations. This is so empowering! Your baby now has a way to start conversations and engage you in his world. As he feels more empowered, your baby also realizes that speaking gives him even more ability to communicate with you and gives him what he needs more quickly. Hence, there is a tendency that babies who sign will learn to speak sooner than their counterparts who do not sign.

Babies who sign make their first sentences (two or more words together) up to six months earlier than babies who do not sign—as early as twelve to fourteen months of age—and they will make three-word sentences up to a year earlier than babies who do not sign. The average child who does not sign makes his first two-word sentence somewhere between eighteen and twenty-four months and three-word sentences somewhere close to three years old.

Here are a few examples of how your signing child's speaking abilities may blossom. At the age of two years, most babies can speak somewhere around fifty words, generally with one or two syllables each. They can put a few two-word or three-word sentences together, such as "I want milk" or "Give ball." When my son was twenty-two months old, he spoke hundreds of words and used complex sentences. I remember one in particular because he used a word I had not taught him. We had been having issues with our car and had told him that the car would be fixed at the "Car Doctor." One day he looked in the garage and noticed the car was missing. He turned around and looked at me and said the following words exactly: "Did Daddy take the car to the *dealership*?" Think about what he said. He used an eight-word sentence with past tense and a huge word–dealership. He must have heard us talking about the dealership and made the connection in his head that this is what the "Car Doctor" was. After I recovered from my amazement, I answered yes, the car was at the dealership.

Another mother, Shannon, explains how her son Eli's learning extends beyond just language to complex thoughts. "Just after Eli's second birthday he called out to me from his room where he had been playing quietly and said, 'Mommy, come here.' When I got there he said, 'I'm standing in an octagon.' Sure enough, he had made an octagon out of eight pencils and was standing in the middle of it! I was impressed and even took a picture." Eli engaged his mother in his world and showed her that at barely two years of age, he could create a complex structure such as an octagon and then let his mother know it.

Some children even begin to speak complex thoughts as early as one year of age. For example, Laura's daughter Fireese is just over one year and she signs more than thirty words and speaks more than twenty words. "She has also started putting words together. She asks for milk and cheerios because we have started giving her cheerios and milk. She still signs while she says the words. It is amazing to see how verbal she is becoming," Laura says. Can you imagine what Fireese is going to be able to say when she is two? It will be much more than the typical two-word sentences of most two-year olds.

The research shows that no delay in language acquisition occurs in children who sign. Ignore your Aunt Betty, who worries that your child will become mute, deaf, or both because you are signing. You are doing an amazing thing for your child, possibly even more amazing than you think.

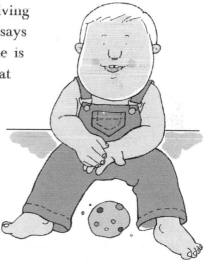

Babies can tell you what they want. This baby wants a cookie.

A Very Important Time for Learning

As parents, we all want our kids to succeed and be smart. We want them to find and make the most of their talents. Recent research shows that in the first three years of life, a baby's brain grows and develops more significantly than at any other concentrated time in his life. This is the time when thinking patterns are established and when development will affect everything a child does for the rest of his life. It is the time when a baby learns how to think, respond, and solve problems. The first three years are a very special opportunity for parents. A baby's brain is twice as active as an adult's brain during these years. This is the most important time for learning and it is also the time when babies have the greatest potential to learn.

Genetics are very important and do influence what skills and abilities your child will have. If you have tendencies toward music or art or science, you may pass these down to your child. New research, however, shows that environment plays an equally important role. Neuroscientists are now finding that the experiences that babies have for the first three years of life impact a baby's brain development greatly. This means that you have an incredible opportunity to meet what nature gives your baby with experiences that will help develop his potential.

A friend of mine wanted to sign with her son after seeing my son's success. But she felt that our results were mostly due to the fact that my son was what she called "really smart"–that he was just naturally advanced. I disagreed with her and asked her to sign with her son and see what happened. To her surprise (but not mine), her son followed almost exactly the same linguistic learning pattern that my son did–nurture at work. He learned to communicate using signs, began to speak words at around fourteen months, learned the alphabet on his own at around eighteen months, was speaking clearly in two- to three-word sentences by twenty months and was linguistically advanced at his second birthday. He also has the same interest in math that my son does and he is learning to read at three years old (the same age at which my son got interested in reading). His speech is so good that he corrects his parents when they make grammatical errors–and that makes us all smile.

I have heard countless similar stories from other parents who have signed with their babies, regardless of educational background. Children who sign have advantages in linguistics because we open the window of communication for them at an earlier time, so they can build more connections in their brains and start the process off better.

Why Signing Works So Well

What is it about signing with your baby that helps children develop more than just an ability to communicate? Parents express that their children who sign tend to be well-adjusted, more even tempered, more polite, and generally better learners. Why? Scientists have shown that certain factors in the first years can help children develop to their full potential. According to the American Academy of Pediatrics, these include the following:

☆ Feeling special and valued
☆ Feeling safe and loved
☆ Knowing what to expect from their environment
☆ Having guidance
☆ Experiencing a balance of freedom and limits
☆ Being exposed to language (and to more than one if possible)
☆ Being exposed to play, exploration, books, music, and age-appropriate toys

Using sign language with your baby will help you do all of these things. The environment you create for your child really does affect him and when you use sign language, you are given extra tools to help facilitate learning and growth in your baby.

Adults are often confused as to how to communicate with a baby and how to create a positive environment in the home and surrounding community. Some parents become very frustrated by the fact that much of the time,

AHA!

Signing with your baby is a multisensory experience that may help the development of both sides of your baby's brain. The left side of the brain is stimulated by the words you say to your baby. The right side of the brain is stimulated by the images your baby sees. When you speak *and* sign together, you are giving your baby input that stimulates both sides of his brain.

they cannot communicate effectively with their baby during a time that is so crucial to development. Lacking an effective way to communicate, some parents give up and stop trying to interact with their child, thinking that they will do this at a later time when their baby is past the "Eat, Sleep, and Poop" stage and is talking.

By interacting with your child in the earliest stages, you can develop communication and language skills, identify developmental problems earlier, create a stimulating environment, and have a positive parenting experience. Your relationship becomes a two-way interaction instead of just a custodial relationship where all you do is make sure your baby is fed and clean. When you sign with your baby, you and your baby participate together in his development. Amazing!

Why signing helps develop your baby's brain

The American Academy of Pediatrics (AAP) suggests that all parents make sure they are doing several specific things to stimulate their baby's brain growth during the first two years of life. When you sign with your baby, you achieve nearly everything the AAP suggests in a simple and effective way. Let's take a look at each AAP suggestion and see how signing works to promote your baby's brain growth.

★ *Provide an environment that is safe and stimulating so that your baby can begin to explore and learn*

When you sign with your baby, you provide visual and auditory stimulation for your child. He is able to interact with you and learn about the world around him.

☆ *Establish a sense of security and well-being with your baby by giving him lots of physical contact and touching*

When you sign with your baby, you have constant physical contact with him. At times, you may direct his hands by placing your hands over his to help him learn to make a sign. You will hold him as you read books together. Because you are directing your attention to your child, you will look at him and talk directly to him. When you sign, you will have more interaction with your baby, which leads to more physical contact and touching.

☆ *Respond to your baby's needs both when he is happy and upset*

Signing gives you a way to let your baby know that you understand his requests—the ones he makes through signing or speaking and the ones you just understand. As early as four months, you can let him know that you understand that he is hungry and wants to eat. He will let you know when he is happy and what he is thinking about.

☆ *Talk and sing to your baby while dressing, feeding, changing, playing, walking, and driving*

Many parents don't know how to talk to someone who cannot talk back. Signing with your baby gives you a way to interact with him and teaches you both how to communicate before your baby can talk. If you are shy about your voice and not sure whether you can sing to your child, don't be. No matter what your voice sounds like, your baby will love it. And if you add signs to your songs, it can be a fun learning experience for both of you.

★ Talk with your baby face-to-face and mimic his sounds

When you sign with your baby, you look at him directly and give him the face- to-face time that he needs to learn more about speaking and communicating.

★ Read every day

Research shows that children who signed as babies read better than their counterparts who do not sign. Signing turns reading into a multisensory experience and gets the hands as well as the ears and eyes engaged in reading. Your baby can participate in the reading process earlier.

★ Speak a second language at home

Using sign language has been shown to have the same effects on the brain as learning any other second language. You are stimulating the parts of the brain that make language acquisition easier.

★ Dance with your baby

Signing may not make you light on your feet, but because you get into a habit of interacting with your baby, activities such as dancing become more commonplace. Dancing and music are important ways to stimulate the brain and provide your child with the basis for later math learning and increased memory skills.

★ Keep stress levels low

One of the biggest stresses for both parents and children is the inability to communicate needs, wants, and desires. Signing gives you both a way to lower frustration levels because you can communicate with each other. This also helps you to keep the stress levels low over the long term.

✪ *Give your baby age-appropriate toys to play with and encourage him to reach for them himself*

Signing adds an additional dimension to play by giving you a way to ask questions and interact with your child during playtime. You not only provide age-appropriate toys, but you also converse and ask questions during playtime, such as "**WHERE** is your airplane?" or "Is your baby **TIRED**? Does she want to go to **BED**?"

✪ *Spend time on the floor with your baby every day*

Signing helps you have a reason to get on the floor, and it gives you a way to interact when you are there. You have a way to discuss your baby's activities with him, ask him questions, and participate in games with him. Because you are signing with your baby, you directly interact with him and have a two-way play time, which is more fulfilling and motivating for both you and your baby.

✪ *Help your baby to learn to sleep for longer periods at night*

Signing can give you a way to discuss with your baby the ritual of going to bed. You can explain that it is time for **SLEEP**. This helps your baby understand the transition to sleep.

✪ *Make sure that other caregivers understand the importance of having a loving bond with your baby*

Caregivers will appreciate being able to communicate with your baby as well. A baby who can sign his needs is easier to take care of than a baby who can only cry and hope that his caregiver can guess his needs. When your caregiver understands that your baby can express himself with a few simple signs, she will probably be happy to learn a few of them.

Signing makes it easier to achieve your parental goals and it helps make your baby's development a much more enjoyable experience for both of you.

But Will My Baby Sign?

Many parents are concerned that their baby will not sign. Even parents who have signed with an older sibling might have doubts that their new baby will sign. Don't worry. All babies are mimics and they want to copy what you are doing. They learn to do everything by watching you, including signing. Your baby will sign to you if you sign to him. As long as your baby is not suffering

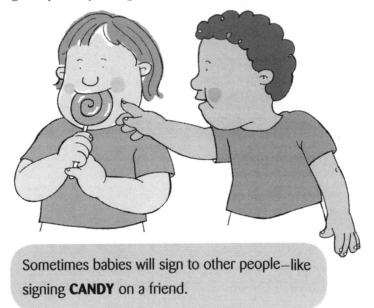

Sometimes babies will sign to other people—like signing **CANDY** on a friend.

from any disabilities or developmental setbacks, his success in signing will have more to do with your willingness to teach him than with anything else. If you are consistent in your signing interactions, your baby should catch on and will sign back when he has the motor skills to do so. Until he has the motor skills, he may respond through grunts or gestures.

If you do have a baby with special needs such as a disease, disability, hospitalization, or other struggle, you will need to be patient. It will take longer, but you can still achieve great results with signing. I have devoted an entire chapter to children with special needs. (See Chapter Eight: Signing with Children Who Have Special Needs.)

If your baby was born premature or near-term (said of a baby born early but not premature), you might want to adapt all dates in this book to his projected gestation date, the date on which he should have been born. Your doctor has probably told you to expect your baby to hit milestones on a schedule based on his gestation date. The same holds true for signing. So, if your baby was two months premature, add two months to the dates when you can expect your baby to sign back and don't give up if he has not made his first sign by seven months. Make sure you are checking for other ways he might be responding to your signs such as grunts, squeals, smiles, and so forth.

AHA!

If you are adopting a baby, signing is a wonderful way to create a bond with your new child. You may be present at your baby's birth and able to introduce him to your family right away. If this is the case, just follow the book chapter by chapter. Or, your baby may come to you from another family or country where customs, language, and interactions are different. Signing can help bridge language and cultural issues and help smooth the transition. It can create a stronger bond between both of you. If you adopt your baby when he is older, or when he has been exposed to another language or to very little language, you will find it easiest to start with the information in Chapter Three: 4–7 Months—I'm Ready to Start. But, you might need to modify the signs you use to include things your baby is interested in or experiences he is having, because he may be more cognitively, physically, and emotionally developed. Be flexible and look to him to see what his interests are.

Experiences of Signing Families

Hundreds of thousands of families have signed with their babies. Some have learned as few as three signs and found that to be effective for them. Most families have learned somewhere between twenty and fifty signs. But others go on to learn many more signs. Here are a few stories from families who are signing with their children.

Jennifer and Alice

Jennifer started signing with her daughter Alice at seven months. She started with **DOG**, **MILK**, **EAT,** and **MORE**. Jennifer first noticed that Alice would nod her head and make grunting noises at about eight or nine months when Jennifer signed **MILK**. Alice made her first sign (**DOG**) at ten months. It took Alice only a month longer to feel comfortable with signing. At fourteen months, she now understands about one hundred signs and signs using about fifty signs.

Jennifer says, "We were at the pool this summer and my daughter Alice had just started signing **BABY**. I wasn't sure what she was doing because she had just started using that sign a few days prior. I said, '**BABY**?' and looked around. Sure enough, about fifty feet away there was a mother nursing her baby. My daughter always looks so pleased when she's made a connection. It's beautiful." Another time, Jennifer and Alice were shopping when Alice began to sign **MILK**. "I was in the middle of a conversation with a friend (a new father himself), but I didn't skip a beat

WOW!

Some limited research has shown that mothers who sign with their babies feel more competent as parents than other mothers. Although there is no scientific backing to say that these mothers *are* more competent, the fact that they feel more comfortable as mothers is a great thing. Being able to communicate with your baby helps you to feel more capable of handling his needs and wants. It also helps you to feel empowered to communicate what you need your baby to know. That is a great start to any relationship!

and handed her the milk. My friend said, 'How did you know what she wanted?' I replied that she had told me and showed him the sign. He just looked shocked." Jennifer says that everyone in the family signs with Alice and this "encourages her to continue learning. Seeing into the window of the baby's mind is amazing!"

Antonette and Christopher

Antonette began signing with Christopher right after he was born. "I began with **MOMMY, DADDY, EAT, MILK,** and **MORE.** Christopher began responding by watching me intently at around three months. When I would sign **MILK** and ask whether he wanted to nurse, he would begin rooting. Even though he first looked at **MILK**, the first sign he actually produced was **MORE** when he was about five months old."

Antonette relates how signing cleared up a language issue for her son at seventeen months: "One day Christopher was playing in his room and heard a noise outside; we went to investigate and found the grounds crew mowing the grass. He asked, 'Car?' I replied, 'No, lawn mower.' He continued to watch out of the window and I realized that he was signing to himself **MORE MORE MORE.** He looked out of the window again, pointed at the machine, and signed **MORE**. I then realized that he was mixing up the word 'more' with 'mower' because they sounded alike to him. I praised him for trying to say what he saw and then showed him the sign for lawn mower." If Antonette had not been able to sign with Christopher, she would never have seen that *more* and *mower* had confused her son. A quick sign and things were straightened out.

Lauri , Megan, and Max

Lauri signs with both her children, Megan and Max. She relates the following about her daughter: "Megan was eleven months when she was sitting in her doll's crib. I told her to come out (I didn't want her to break it), but she insisted. Then I said to her 'It's for your baby doll.' Then, she looked at me and shook her head and signed **BOAT**. She was pretending it was a boat.

At her young age, she was *pretending* and I was able to play with her instead of ruining it for her. I got a box and we continued to play **BOAT**." Being able to sign with Megan gave Lauri a way to understand what her daughter was really doing and let her respond in a way that gave both of them what they needed.

Lauri's son Max also benefits from signing. When Max was twelve months old, Lauri had the following experience: "Max was trying to get a lid off a jar. He looked at me and signed **HELP** and showed me the jar. I asked what he wanted with it; he signed **HAT** and then pointed to the lid. He was able to use the limited signs he knew to get his point across that he wanted the lid off the jar. Using the sign **HAT** let him communicate with me instead of throwing the jar at me in a fit (his usual reaction of frustration)."

Thalia, Lance, and Trinity

Thalia is a mother to twenty-month old twins, Lance and Trinity. Twins tend to talk late because they can create their own "language" to communicate with each other. Also, because there are two babies, people tend to talk to both of them rather than directly to one or the other. Thalia says, "It was my hope that teaching them to sign would allow them to communicate with me sooner and that I wouldn't have to wait for them to begin verbal communication to understand what they were saying. I first began signing with them at six months, I started with **MORE**, **DIAPER**, and **EAT**. After a couple of months I gave up. When I started back up again around the middle of their 11th month, I added **ALL DONE**, **HAT**, **MOM**, and **DAD**.

Trinity began to pick it up immediately. It was almost as if something had been unlocked for her. She signed back within a few weeks. She signed **MORE** and then **ALL DONE** followed the very next day. Once she started signing, she just couldn't be stopped. Now she understands hundreds of signs, and she signs using 100 to 130 signs. Lance liked signing immediately as well, but he had no desire to sign back to me until he signed **AIRPLANE** at fourteen months old. Anytime he saw or heard an airplane, he was quick to make that sign. He also signed **AIRPLANE** when he saw helicopters, leaf blowers, and lawn mowers. He didn't sign anything else until he was sixteen months old, but he signed **AIRPLANE** a lot. Now Lance recognizes probably one hundred signs, but he signs only around fifty to seventy signs."

Tami, Kenny, and Sean

Tami is a mother of ten children, six of whom are under six years old. She is especially grateful for signing with her two boys. "My twin boys did not talk, so I started teaching them signs when they were three. Kenny learned to talk using sign and words. But Sean did not sign as well because he has fine motor issues and severe Apraxia. He now has been in speech therapy for two years and he is progressing in language. Sean still uses signs when he speaks and he often communicates with just signs. Signing saved us by creating a bridge across the frustration of not being able to communicate with words."

Joelle and Cecelia

Joelle has been signing with her daughter for about two years. At twenty-eight months, Cecelia signs more than five hundred signs, as well as the alphabet and numbers. "When she was a baby, we started with first signs such as **MILK**, **EAT**, and **MORE**. As both her signing vocabulary and ours increased, we added signs for whatever she was interested in at the time. When we taught her colors, we added the signs of colors. When we visited the zoo, we added animal signs and so forth. The more we add, the more she uses.

"Signing is a blessing and I continue to sign with her even though she speaks in complete sentences such as 'I'm hot. Can you turn down the heat please,' because she is now learning to spell and read. She has known her letters since seventeen months and has known the letter sounds since she was two. She now tries to sound out words when we read and when we play with her bath letters, we say words and try to spell them. All this happened thanks to signing (and my genius kid!)." Although Cecelia's abilities are extraordinary, they are common among children who sign with their parents as babies.

Kim and Gage

Kim, who is a speech language pathologist, began signing with her younger son, Gage, when he was about eight months old. "Our first family picture shows him approximating the sign for **MORE** (he was about nine months old) because the photographer was using a squeaky puppet to make the boys smile. When Gage was about twenty-two months old, he hadn't yet progressed to using words. I had been worried for a while, but all my family and friends kept telling me to wait and said, 'You know too much; you are too close to it.' Our older son talked late, but he began with sentences. He went from no words to more than fifty words and phrases between fifteen and eighteen months. He continued to talk above expectation. Gage was the second child, with an older brother who did stuff for him and wouldn't shut up, so I decided to wait a bit longer. He babbled loads and used more than three hundred signs, even three- to four-word phrases, so I decided to have him evaluated by a colleague.

"I thought he might have a problem with the muscles in his mouth. Sure enough my fears were confirmed and he was diagnosed as apraxic (a motor coordination disorder that affects speech skills). Gage remained unintelligible for another six or so months. At about two and a half years he got to the point where some people, other than me, his dad, and my mom, could understand him. Even though through the whole process he couldn't use words to tell us what he wanted or needed, he did sign. I can't imagine how we would have gotten through it without sign. You just never know when it will be 'a neat thing to do' versus a tool that will be needed for a child's development. We still sign today for literacy, reading skills, behavior management, and songs—and we all love it."

Enjoy the Journey

Throughout this book, you will see how signing has helped families such as yours create better bonds with their children and enhance the communication between parent and child. In each chapter you will learn how your baby is developing and what signs to use at each age. You will learn which activities you want to sign about first and why signing works so well with these activities. Because this book is synchronized to your baby's development, you will be able to focus your signing interactions to achieve the greatest effectiveness. Signing with your child is truly an amazing experience that you don't want to miss. It can enhance your relationship with your baby and give both of you a more successful way to communicate. Enjoy the journey!

[i] *Caring for Your Baby and Young Child*, Revised Edition: Birth to Age 5 by American Academy of Pediatrics and "Speech and language development milestones" Mayo Clinic.com

[ii] M.E. Anthony, R. Lindert, *Signing Smart with Babies and Toddlers* (St. Martins 2005)

[iii] M.E. Anthony, R. Lindert, *Signing Smart with Babies and Toddlers* (St. Martins 2005)

[iv] S. Goodwyn, L. Acredolo, and C. Brown, "Impact Of Symbolic Gesturing On Early Language Development," *Journal of Non-Verbal Behavior* 24 (2000):81–103

[v] L. Nicolosi, E. Harryman, J Kresheck, *Terminology of Communication Disorders* (Lippincott Williams & Wilkins; 5th edition October 1, 2003)

[vi] S. Goodwyn, L. Acredolo, and C. Brown, "Impact Of Symbolic Gesturing On Early Language Development," *Journal of Non-Verbal Behavior* 24 (2000):81–103

[vii] L. Nicolosi, E. Harryman, J Kresheck, *Terminology of Communication Disorders* (Lippincott Williams & Wilkins; 5th edition October 1, 2003)

[viii] Acredolo, L. P., & Goodwyn, S.W. (July 2000). "The long-term impact of symbolic gesturing during infancy on IQ at age 8," Paper presented at the meetings of the International Society for Infant Studies, Brighton, UK.

Note: The Zero to Three website is a great resource to help you know what your baby should be doing during the first three years of life. Go to www.zerotothree.org.

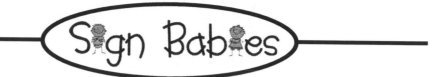
Chapter Two

Birth to Three Months– I'm Just Not Ready Yet, But . . .

Parents often ask when they should begin signing with their babies. Any time is fine. However, some times are more effective than others. For example, when your baby is very young (from birth to three months generally), her eyesight is not well developed. When she is one month old, she can see clearly only at a distance of eight to twelve inches and she prefers black-and-white or high contrast images.

By the age of four months, however, your baby will change greatly and will go from being a newborn–totally dependent on you–to a baby who can control more of her responses. She'll also start interacting with you. Even though you might decide to sit it out and not sign during the first three months, there are some things you should know about your baby's development. You should know how to interact with your baby at this time, which will help you with your communication later.

In this chapter, we'll take a look at the following:

✫ How your baby is developing during the first three months

✫ How you should be communicating with your baby during the first three months

✫ When you should start signing

✫ What to do if your baby will be with another caregiver

The First Three Months, A.K.A., The Fourth Trimester

The first three months are crucial, so don't make the mistake of thinking that nothing very important is going on because your baby seems to be interested only in food, sleep, and clean diapers (what we call in our house the "eat, sleep, poop stage"). Actually, this is a time when you can focus on creating a bond with your baby through proximity. If you have the opportunity to be at home with your baby, take it. Tremendous bonding takes place in the wee hours of the morning and during sessions of rocking and cuddling during the day. If you are unable to be at home, hold and love your baby as much as you can. In any case, don't equate your baby's inability to communicate with an inability to understand your love. What you do now sets the stage for your child's feelings of security and trust.

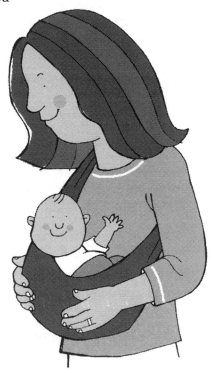

Some doctors and researchers have suggested that the first three months of your baby's life ought to be thought of as a fourth trimester. Dr. Harvey Karp, pediatrician and author of the book *Happiest Baby on the Block*, suggests that due to evolutionary tradeoffs, human babies are born sooner than they are ready to face the world. Because humans have large brains but are born to parents with small pelvic bones (thanks to our ability to walk upright), a tradeoff had to be made: babies had to be born earlier. He suggests that several cultures intuitively understand this fourth trimester concept and spend the first three months carrying babies constantly and giving them a womblike experience. It is true that many cultures around the world revere the first ninety days of a baby's life as a very sacred time for the baby to stay close to the mother. In some cultures, women do little or no housework during this time, relying on relatives to help as they spend the time feeding and nurturing the newborn. In other cultures, babies are carried in a sling where they can be nursed at will by their mother and are located close to her heart, hearing the sounds they heard in the womb.

Whether or not you have the chance to stay home, the transition of becoming a new parent can be difficult. Issues of depression, isolation, and so forth may make this time less than ideal. Make the most of the time you have with your baby at this time by creating the best relationship you can. The greatest way to do this is to embrace the experience you will have with your baby and appreciate her new life. She is an amazing creation. She has so much to learn and so much to share with you. Watch her, hold her, talk to her, and share your thoughts with her. She may not be able to understand your words, but she will understand that you are reaching out to her. You can also learn to give her a baby massage. Massaging your baby is a wonderful way to connect with her. All of your interactions with her lay the foundation for your relationship with her in the future.

Let's take a closer look at how your baby develops during the first three months.

Motor development

Your baby's arm movements develop rapidly. Her hands will be clasped tightly. You will be able to open her fingers and place a rattle in her hand. Although, she will automatically grasp the rattle, she will not be able to move it to her mouth. By the end of this time, your baby will be able to relax her hand and it will be open about half the time. If you place a rattle in her hand, she will be able to bring it to her face and explore it. You may also find your baby staring at her hands for long periods of time towards the end of the first three months. She may be able to raise her hand to her mouth by the third month.

During the fourth month, she is likely to learn to place her thumb inside her mouth (many parents abhor the idea that their baby might suck their thumb, but this movement is a significant motor skill development). During the third or fourth month, she will also get her whole arm movement coordinated and will be able to reach out for things like toys swinging overhead.

Visual development

Your baby's vision starts out with the ability to clearly see only those objects that are eight to twelve inches from her face. She will focus on one thing and not see the big picture. She cannot track movement very well. However, by the age of two months, things will improve dramatically. She will see your whole face instead of just focusing on your eyes and she will track your movements. By the end of the first three months, she will become more interested in her environment and will spend time focusing on objects such as her hands or your face. She may also be able to move her head and track your movement across the room, as her distance vision is also improving rapidly. She can now smile at you too.

Hearing development

During this time, your baby's hearing will also improve. If your baby was not tested for hearing at birth, you should make sure that your pediatrician checks her hearing now. If your baby has any hearing issues, this is the most crucial time to find that out. Babies who are hearing impaired should be identified as soon as possible, so that both parents and children can get the help they need. If babies are deprived of language at these early stages—whether it's spoken language in the case of hearing babies or sign language in the case of deaf babies—their ability to learn can be greatly delayed.

One of the benefits of signing early with babies that I often hear from mothers of hearing impaired children is that they had established signing as a language before they knew that their child had a hearing problem. Karen, for example, has signed with her four children. She started signing with her first daughter at three and then signed with the other three children from birth. Later, she found out that her youngest daughter, Kara, is deaf. Karen started with the same signs for all her kids: **MILK, MOMMY, MORE,** and **DADDY**. Because Kara was able to learn language at an early age, she is developing language at the same rate as other children. Whereas many hearing impaired children are delayed in their language learning because they are not diagnosed until they are one year or older.

Language development

For hearing babies, a parent's voice is the most wonderful sound. A baby tends to respond to her mother's high-pitched voice. This may be the reason why we associate baby talk with high-pitched sounds. Have you seen big burly men talking in high-pitched voices with babies? Maybe we know intuitively that this is the sound babies like most.

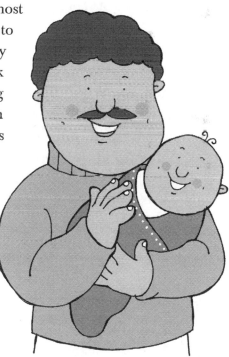

By one month, your baby will be able to distinguish your voice from other sounds, even if you are in another room. By two months, your baby may begin to "talk" with you by making basic cooing sounds. This is the beginning of the "conversation" because your baby is learning the importance of communication and speech. She will learn many of the subtle rules of conversation, such as taking turns, tone, and speed and pacing of a conversation. During this time your baby will smile when she hears your voice, begin to babble and imitate some sounds, and turn her head toward sounds she hears.

Recent research in the United States and Australia shows that your baby is also communicating with you through her cries. Priscilla Dunstan, a mom from Australia, says she's unlocked the secret language of babies. Dunstan has a gift for deciphering sounds that she used to understand her baby, Tom. "I was able to pick out certain patterns in his cries and then remember what those patterns were later on when he cried again." Then Dunstan realized that other babies were saying the same "words" through their cries. After testing her baby language theory on more than one thousand infants around the world, Dunstan says there are five sound reflexes that all babies from birth to three months old say:

Neh = I'm hungry

Owh = I'm sleepy (like a yawn)

Heh = I'm experiencing discomfort

Eair = I have lower gas

Eh = I need to burp

Dunstan explains, "Babies all around the world have the same reflexes, and they therefore make the same sounds." If parents don't respond to those reflexes, Dunstan says, the baby will eventually stop using them. Listen for these sounds in your baby's precry (before she starts crying hysterically). Dunstan has created a DVD to help parents learn to hear the different sounds their babies are making. For more on the research done in Australia and in the United States at Brown University, see the website at www.dunstanbaby.com.

Whether or not you are able to discern your baby's cries, you are only a few months away from two-way conversations with your baby. How you interact with her now will help your baby develop her communication abilities down the road.

Communicating with Your Baby from Birth to Three Months

Even during the first three months, babies are very receptive to your talking them through daily activities. Babies differentiate sounds very early and can figure out how words begin and end. They can also distinguish different inflections as early as six months.

As you are nursing or feeding, have a conversation with your baby. Do this only during daylight hours so that your baby does not become overstimulated at night when you want her to learn to go to sleep. When you go to bathe your baby, tell her you are going to give her a bath. You can even describe the process you are going through as you do it. "Sadie, we are going to take a bath now. See, here is your bathtub. The water is warm and the soap smells good. Do you like having your head scrubbed? Now we are going to rinse you off and take you out of the tub. Doesn't this dry, warm towel feel nice?" You get the picture.

Some parents feel very awkward having this one-sided conversation. However, talking with your baby now forms a critical foundation for your baby's communication skills and for your signing experience. Later we will discuss how you can use "parallel talk" and "self-talk" to increase your child's language experiences.

You can vary your conversations by singing and reading books to your baby. You can sing your favorite Top-Ten songs or children's songs. Some parents decide early on that they will never listen to children's music and will

AHA!

What if you don't speak with your baby? Speech language pathologists suggest that not speaking with your baby could be setting her up for linguistic problems in the future. The more you speak with your baby, the better chance she has to learn to speak well. Signing helps you achieve this effectively because you speak directly in your child's line of sight while you sign. She not only hears you, but she sees what your face and mouth are doing—great clues to learning language.

expose their baby only to "real" music. They may be missing out, however, as most children's music has simple rhythms and rhymes that teach children valuable verbal skills. Reading books also helps develop language skills in your baby. Pick up classics such as *Goodnight, Moon,* and *Pat the Bunny,* but don't be afraid to read the newspaper or adult reading-level books to your child as well.

By varying the types of books you read, you expose your baby to all the rhythms of language. If you have older children, this is a great time to create bonds between your children. You can hold your baby while reading to your older children. If your children are old enough to read, have them read to your baby as well.

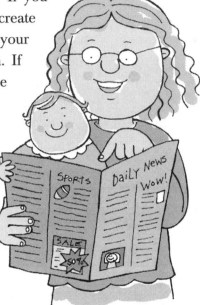

If you speak with your baby during the day for the first three months, you are getting yourself in the habit of creating communication opportunities. When your baby is ready to see you sign at about four months old, you are already in a communication routine. All you need to do is add signs to your conversations. Your baby will get used to your conversations and will notice that you are also doing something with your hands—the same thing each time she takes a bath, for example. She will quickly begin to associate the signs with the language sounds and with the activity. This is the beginning of the conversation.

Respond to your baby's needs

Some parents worry that they are going to spoil their child by responding to her needs. A consensus of recent research and wisdom is that this is not the case during the first six months of life. Rather, responding to your baby's needs instills a feeling of security and acceptance in your child. In fact, the American Academy of Pediatrics suggests that responding to your baby's needs promptly will help your baby learn a sense of independence, which will *decrease* her neediness in the future and foster a healthy, strong sense of independence. Additionally, what could be more loving and reassuring than teaching her to communicate her needs so that those needs can be met?

Smile!

Another milestone that your baby will reach during the first three months is the first smile. Generally some time after the first month, your baby will make her first voluntary smile. Your baby will soon learn that moving her lips is a conversation starter and will get you to interact with her. When you see that smile, you can't help but start talking and praising your baby. She will feel good about the interaction and smile more. This leads you to even more conversation, and as your baby begins to make sounds, she will coo and babble to continue the conversation, eliciting more responses and interactions from you.

Babies will often try to engage you in a smile conversation. Sometimes, you will find your baby trying to get your attention by smiling at you. Respond to her by smiling back and start conversing. When you smile back, she will often respond with a

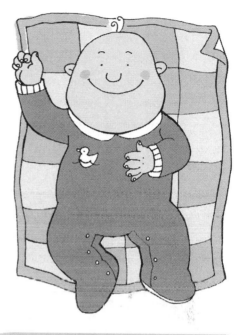

TWO CENTS

Parents want to meet their children's needs and have happy babies. However, remember that every baby comes with her own disposition. During the first three months of life, you will learn a lot about your baby's disposition and her likes and dislikes. Don't feel frustrated if you didn't get one of those rare happy, content babies. Embrace your baby's personality.

whole body smile—her arms and legs will get into the act of communicating. She understands that you two are communicating with each other. Enjoy these times and use them to teach your baby that she is loved and cared for. Talk to her and interact with her often. The first three years are the most important time in your baby's brain development and the more interaction she has with you in smile conversation, the more developed her brain will be—even at this early age.

TWO CENTS

One great way to build a relationship of trust with your baby is to learn infant massage. Infant massage has been practiced by other cultures for centuries. The medical community has studied the benefits of massage on both full-term and pre-term babies and found that massage relaxes infants, enhances bonding, aids in growth and development, improves sleep, and promotes communication. Parents who massage their babies become more aware of their baby's nonverbal cues, and the babies in turn learn to trust that their parents will take care of their needs. Creating this relationship helps prepare your baby for signing.

Should You Start Signing Now?

Because you have decided to sign with your baby, you must be wondering how this will affect your interaction with your baby. You might be surprised to learn that when you sign you will probably talk with your baby more than you would if you did not sign. It may seem like a paradox at first, so let me explain. Parents who sign with their baby, intentionally engage their baby in conversation. They make a conscious choice to explain to their baby that they are going to change the baby's diaper or give the baby a bath. Many nonsigning parents do these activities without explaining to their baby what they are doing or why. Or, they speak to their baby with their back turned. Parents who sign face their babies so that their babies can see their lips and hear their voices more clearly, both of which help babies learn to speak.

The choice to sign with your baby should be based more on your state of mind rather than on your effectiveness. If you are feeling stressed out, tired, or otherwise not yourself, don't worry about signing yet. Babies are developing their visual acuity at this time and their motor skills are limited. What this means is that your baby probably won't see much of your attempts to communicate and won't be able to sign back. So, relax and just hold and hug your baby. Talk with her, let her know how much you love her. The more low-stress environment you can give her, the better.

The bonding you can do with your baby at this age is more important than signing. When I was a first-time mom, I used to read books that told me not to worry about the dishes in the sink and the mess on the floor and just embrace my baby. That was hard for me to do because I felt that I had to get everything done like I used to. I have since learned that the wonderful, close time of the first three months goes by so fast. No one remembers that the dishes didn't get done or that you ate takeout and frozen foods. What does come from this time is a feeling of security and trust for your baby and a feeling for you that you are going to be a good parent. Relax and enjoy your baby and the time you have together—no matter how much it is.

What If My Baby Will Be Cared for By Someone Else?

Many parents return to the workforce and are worried about how the primary caregiver will react to the idea of signing with your baby. If your baby's primary caregiver is older, like a grandparent, be prepared for some scoffing. You might hear things like, "In our day we never signed with babies and we got along just fine." Or if the caregiver has more than one child to take care of, she might be reluctant and claim that she doesn't have time to learn signs. And besides, she'll tell you, she is not signing with the other children. She may say that signing will be too much pressure. Even though your baby might be too young now to start signing, consider letting your caregiver know now that you intend to sign with your baby and hope that she participates.

There are a few ways to approach the situation with your caregiver. You could give her this book and ask her to read it—especially "Chapter One:

What Is Baby Sign Language." She may become convinced after reading it that signing has made a difference in the lives of other families. There are often local and national news reports on the effectiveness of signing with hearing babies. You can even show her clips on signing on the Internet. If you have friends who have signed with their children, ask them to talk to her about their personal experience or let her watch their interactions with their child. Video clips of babies signing are available on the Sign Babies website at www.signbabies.com. Or you can listen to me talk about baby sign language on my weekly radio show and podcasts on Babies and Moms: Birth and Beyond. There are great discussions of signing there each week and videos to help parents. Go to www.babiesandmomsradio.com.

IMPORTANT: Be careful to not ask any child who can sign to "perform" a sign. Children should never be asked to sign as a performance, as this is an unnatural request and will not be successful. If you want to demonstrate a child's signing abilities, place that child in a situation where she will sign naturally. For example, ask her if she wants an apple. She will sign **APPLE** to reply in the affirmative.

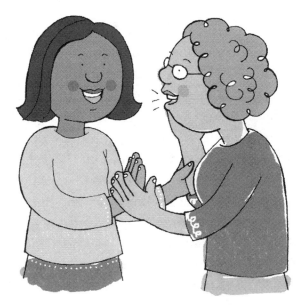

A caregiver's reluctance to sign with your baby may stem from fears that she has to learn a whole new language to sign with your child. Alleviating these fears may solve your problem. If you explain that you will be teaching your baby a limited number of signs, this might help. You can even limit the number of signs your caregiver will use to as few as five to ten signs. Although it would be optimal if your caregiver would learn more signs, even a very few signs will help both your baby and her caregiver. This approach often also works well with fathers who are reluctant to sign with their children or grandparents who think this is just a fad.

Ashley nannied for two young girls, Lily and Cara. The older, Lily, was adopted from China when she was almost one year old. Cara was born exactly one month after Lily arrived in the United States. Their mother returned to work as a neonatologist five weeks after Cara was born. Ashley explains, "When Lily first came to the States, Anna and her husband were adamant about teaching her to sign. When I started working for them full-time, I thought that this concept was absolutely absurd. I couldn't understand how a Chinese girl that couldn't walk at the age of one would be able to sign for things that she needed or wanted. Soon after that, we were signing consistently using approximately three different signs: **BANANA**, **MORE**, and **MILK**. Those seemed to be the 'lifeblood' of our relationship and I couldn't believe how much they helped. Even when Lily learned to communicate somewhat clearly, her speech was delayed until she was about eighteen months old. We would still use signing as a means of communication. I am a firm believer in signing and as soon as I am a mother, I will also use the same method."

If your attempts to persuade your child's primary caregiver to sign with your baby fail, you can still be successful in signing with your baby. You will be the primary source of signing when you are together. It may take more time for your baby to sign back, but when you demonstrate that your baby does communicate using signs, often caregivers give in and learn a few signs.

Lauri had to return to work soon after her daughter Alexa was born. She entrusted the care of her daughter to her mother-in-law for several hours a day. Lauri began signing with Alexa when she was six months old and discussed this with her mother-in-law who immediately refused to sign with her granddaughter. At first, Lauri was disappointed, but decided to keep signing when she was with Alexa. "It was hard because we did not have a lot of time together and I felt like Alexa was not seeing enough sign for it to matter. Her grandmother would not sign with her at all. It took Alexa longer to sign back, but when she was about twelve months old, she began signing with me. Her first sign was **MORE**. She wanted more cereal. I was so shocked when I saw her sign the first time.

Over the next few months, she began to sign more often and use more signs. She would also sign to her grandmother, but her grandmother didn't know what she was doing. One day, my mother-in-law asked why Alexa tapped her fingers together. When I told her that meant she wanted more of something, my mother-in-law was amazed. Since then, she has learned three or four signs that help her with Alexa. She won't learn more than that, but Alexa and I are fine with it. We still sign at home and Alexa now knows about twenty-five signs."

Helping your caregiver learn the signs

When you do begin signing with your baby at four to seven months, your caregiver might be frustrated that she does not understand the signs your baby is making (your baby will generally sign back some time between seven to twelve months). Let her know now that you plan to sign with your baby and involve her as much as she feels comfortable. Teach her the signs as your baby learns them. Leave a visual cue for your caregiver as well. Many parents find that leaving the *Sign Babies ASL Flash Cards* for the signs they are working on with their baby helps the caregiver learn and recognize the signs too. Your caregiver might start learning just because she is forced by your baby's need to be understood. This can also happen in reverse and parents can be pushed by what the caregiver learns and teaches.

Trisha is a nanny who started signing with the twin babies she cares for at a young age. "Finally, when they were around nine months old, they started signing back. The parents thought it was cool, but didn't make any serious attempt to learn it themselves. However, now the babies, sixteen months old, have started signing so many things that the parents don't understand. I'm showing the babies something *once* and they are incorporating it into their repertoire! The parents are realizing now that they need to get on board so the babies don't get frustrated. I'm starting to stay late to tutor the adults and am leaving lots of flash cards for them to study on their own. It's so amazing to have this extra window into the minds of the children!"

If your caregiver is resistant, take it slow and don't push it. Sometimes your baby can change her mind. Many grandparents and caregivers have begun signing after they saw a baby signing. If your caregiver decides not to sign with your baby, it does not mean that your baby will not sign with you. Besides, you have a few months until your baby starts to sign. With time, your caregiver's opinion might change.

Summary

In this chapter, we discussed:

- ☆ The first three months are like a fourth trimester. Your baby is adjusting to being outside the womb.
- ☆ Take time to bond with your baby. This is an important time to create a sense of security for your baby and a sense that you will be able to be a good parent.
- ☆ Your baby can only see clearly 8-12 inches away from her face at birth, but will be able to see you across the room by the end of the third month.
- ☆ Your baby responds to your voice and may "talk" back to you by the end of the third month.
- ☆ You can help your baby learn the rules of language by talking, singing, and reading.
- ☆ If your baby will be cared for by someone else, discuss with them your desire to sign with your baby and explain how it can help them and your baby bond and communicate.

Bottom Line

Relax and enjoy your new baby. Your love is the most important thing your baby can receive from you right now. You can start to sign with your baby, but she might not see your efforts. By the fourth month, your baby will be ready to watch you sign.

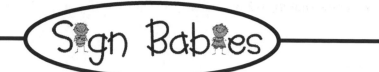

Chapter Three

Four to Seven Months— I'm Ready to Start

At four months, your baby is ready for you to start signing with him. You must be noticing that your baby at age four months is a vastly different baby than he was at birth. He can now see you across the room and can interact with you as well. If you talk to him, he coos and smiles. He is watching how you communicate and is learning the subtle rules of language. Even though it may be several months until your baby signs back to you, he is ready to have you add signs to your conversations. Most babies sign back somewhere between seven and ten months, but they will respond to your signs in other ways that let you know the message is coming through loud and clear.

In this chapter, we'll take a look at the following:

☆ How your baby is developing from four to seven months

☆ How to start signing with your baby

☆ What signs to start signing with your baby

Note: All babies are developmentally unique. You know your baby better than anyone. Take things at his pace. If he is ready sooner, then speed up, or if he seems to take a laid back approach, you should too. If he was premature, you might need to adjust everything to his gestation date and not expect him to sign as soon as other babies. Or if he has another developmental issue, you might need to adapt things even more. Chapter Eight: Signing with Children with Special Needs discusses several developmental issues and recommends how to modify signing with special needs children to suit their specific issues.

Your Baby's Development

Right now your baby is learning to coordinate his senses of touch, vision, and hearing. His motor skills are increasing as well. He is learning to grasp, roll over, sit up, and may even be crawling by the end of this period.

In addition to the increases in sensory and physical coordination, your baby now has more ability to choose his own actions and reactions. He will learn to pick up and explore a toy, or he may cry because he wants to change activities. He will become more interactive and might become a show-off, smiling and playing with anyone. This is the period when your baby's personality really begins to blossom. It is also a key time to start signing with your baby. Because your baby is becoming more alert and more interested in the world around him, he is primed for watching and learning from you.

Every day with your baby will be a new adventure as he gains new skills and explores his personality. Even if this is not your first child, your relationship will be different because your baby is different. Embrace this exciting reality and enjoy the experience. Signing will help you learn more about your baby and see into his thoughts and personality.

Motor development

During this period, your baby gains greater control over his body. He is learning to sit up, roll over, and use his hands to grasp. Your baby does not have the manual dexterity to make very many signs at this age and may not have the control to make distinctive signs until he is seven to nine months old. But it is not uncommon for parents who start to sign with their babies at around four months to see their babies attempt to make a sign back. Generally, babies will sign **MILK** or **MORE** as their first sign. If your baby does not attempt to sign, don't worry. Babies who can't yet get their hands together to sign will respond in other ways–some even very amusing. My son, for example, panted when I asked him if he wanted milk or when I made the sign for **MILK**. A friend's son squealed in delight when his mother would sign **MILK**.

Visual development

Your baby's eyesight is also increasing and will continue to expand until about seven months. Now, he can see clearly several feet in front of his eyes and can track faster and faster movements. He can now follow a ball as it rolls across the room, is stimulated by a mobile, and enjoys more complex patterns and movements. Adding signing to the conversation you have had with your baby since birth adds visual interest and fascination to your interactions.

TWO CENTS

If your baby does not seem to be interested in the shapes, colors, or objects you introduce, or if one or both his eyes turn in or out, talk to your pediatrician. This is an important time to catch visual issues that may be able to be corrected.

Language development

In addition to physical development, this is a great time of language development for your baby. Previously, your baby was interested in your tone, pitch, and voice level. Now, he begins to distinguish individual sounds. He begins to hear how these sounds combine into words and sentences. Your baby can recognize his name. When you call to him, he will turn his head toward you. He will also recognize the names of the people he associates with most–mommy,

AHA!

Some moms who sign with their hearing babies are reporting that their babies move their fingers in a kind of finger babble much like their vocal babble. This is common among both hearing and deaf children of deaf parents. If your baby babbles with his hands or his voice, it is a sign that he is processing language and taking steps forward. So, look for finger babble and also verbal babble!

daddy, brother, and so forth. Your baby will also start to babble during this time. Interestingly, babies babble in the same rhythmic pattern of their native language. Hearing and deaf babies of deaf parents will begin to babble in sign language using their fingers to babble, because this is often the primary language in the home.

Listen closely to your baby's babbling and you will recognize that your baby is working out linguistic characteristics. He will raise and drop his voice as if he is asking a question or making a statement. You can reinforce this by picking up on the sounds your baby is working on, and building on the conversation with both sounds and signs. If your baby is making the sound "mah," you can sign and say, "You sound like you are saying **MOM** (make the sign for mom when you say it). I am so glad you want to say **MOM.** Mom, mom, mom, mom (sign **MOM** repeatedly)."

It becomes increasingly important to engage your baby in linguistic learning as you near the end of the four to seven month period. The time from six to nine months is generally when your baby actively imitates the sounds of speech and is a time when he feels the need to express himself even more strongly. The American Academy of Pediatrics suggests that some of the best words to introduce your baby to during four to seven months are simple syllable words such as:

baby
cat
dog
go

hot

cold

milk

eat

walk

mama

dad

It should not surprise you that many of these words are the best words to sign with your baby.

Cognitive development

Your baby's cognitive abilities are growing by leaps and bounds. His attention span and memory are increasing. He is learning the concept of cause and effect and will undoubtedly spend a lot of time experimenting with this. When baby repeatedly drops a spoon and mom repeatedly picks it up, what parent hasn't wondered when this cause and effect game will end, only to have it repeated over and over again.

By the end of four to seven months, your baby will also begin to understand that things exist even when he cannot see them (which may be a reason why your baby cries when you leave the room). This is called *object permanence.* Your baby's understanding that things exist that he cannot see will also help him to find partially hidden objects. This is a

TWO CENTS

Your baby should have been tested for hearing at birth. But if you notice that your baby does not babble or repeat sounds by the end of this period, discuss it with your pediatrician at your six-month appointment. If your baby has had frequent ear infections, he could have fluid in his inner ear that is interfering with his hearing. Or, he may have another physical issue that can be addressed at this time. If your pediatrician cannot diagnose a problem, ask for a referral to a children's hearing specialist for a second opinion.

good time to start playing peek-a-boo or hiding games. Later, we will discuss how to use object permanence to introduce signs to your baby.

Social development

Accompanying the other changes that happen in this period, your baby may experience a dramatic emergence of his personality. At the beginning of this period, he may seem very passive, but toward the end, your baby may become much more assertive—showing the stuff he is really made of. As he gains more physical and cognitive abilities, he becomes more eager to reach out and interact with the world around him, especially with you and other caregivers. He may become a bit more demanding of your attention as you are the most interesting thing and the best teacher he has. This interest makes the period starting at about six months a stellar time to sign with your baby. Your baby enjoys social play and responding to others—excellent conditions for introducing more sign.

Let's Get Signing!

As a parent, my favorite time with my babies starts during this period. Some parents are huge fans of the newborn stage, but I really love and embrace the blossoming of my children into individuals with personalities—personalities that want to communicate with me. This is also the time when babies begin to do things such as play, eat, and move. Because your baby is interacting more than ever, you have more topics to "discuss."

For example, think of all the things you will be able to sign with your baby as he learns to eat. Your signing experience might be like this: "Do you want to **EAT**? Yum. I have some **BANANA** for you. Do you want **MORE BANANA**? Ok. We are **ALL DONE** with the **BANANA**. Do you want some **MILK**?" This is simplified, but you can see how many words you can sign with your baby during the act of eating.

Start simple

You are ready to start signing with your baby. He is in the prime age to see you signing. Start with five to ten signs. You will want to choose a few signs for things you need and a few signs for things your baby is interested in. To make it easier for you to remember the signs and incorporate them in to what you do, think about them in relation to the activities in which you will be using them. Some of the signs that are best to start with are listed below by activity. Many of the signs can be used in more than one situation.

Note: Signs indicated with asterisks are the ones you should start with at four months. Because there is a huge developmental difference between babies at four and seven months, you may not need some of these signs until six or seven months. For example, most babies do not begin to eat solid foods until they are six months old, so some of the meal signs may not yet apply.

Meal signs
- **MILK***
- **ALL DONE/FINISHED***
- **MORE***
- **EAT**
- **YES**

Diaper/Dressing signs
- **CHANGE DIAPERS***
- **CLOTHES**
- **ALL DONE***
- **LIGHT or FAN***
- **UP**
- **MASSAGE**

Activity signs
- **BOOK***
- **ALL DONE/FINISHED***

- **MORE***
- **PLAY**
- **MUSIC**
- **CAR**
- **DOG/CAT**
- **BEAR**
- **YES**

Bath signs
- **BATH***
- **ALL DONE/FINISHED**

Bedtime signs
- **BOOK***
- **SLEEP or BED***
- **MUSIC**
- **BEAR**

These signs are effective because:

☆ They are distinct. Each sign looks different than the other sign so there is no way to confuse them.

☆ They relate to the things your baby is doing.

☆ They can be used in situations that occur often during the day.

Whether you choose five or ten signs to start with is not as important as choosing signs that interest your baby and that you will use often.

Each of these signs will be discussed later in the chapter, with an explanation of when to make them and illustrations of how to sign them. Let's first discuss the entire process of signing with your baby so you know how to incorporate these signs into your daily activities.

Sign in context

You never need to make a specific time for signing. Just incorporate signing into whatever you are doing with your baby. This allows you to make the signs in the proper context so your baby can associate the sign with the activity. This means that you should show the sign while you are interacting with the concept or object. For example, you can sign **MILK** while feeding your baby a bottle or while nursing. Or, if your baby has begun eating, sign **EAT** while your baby eats.

IMPORTANT: Babies live in the here and now. They are just beginning to conceptualize things that are not present and will not have a good grasp on this concept until the end of this period in their development. This is especially true for activities. So, don't confuse them by signing something that is not "here and now" for them. For example, don't try to explain to them that you are going to read a book in thirty minutes. If you say "We are going to read a **BOOK**," make sure you are ready to do it now. Your baby won't understand that he has to wait for it.

AHA!

Sign Babies ASL Flash Cards are a great way to learn the signs while you are introducing them to your child. They include the same signs as this book, along with wonderful illustrations of the people, objects, and emotions you and your baby need to know. The cards were designed for the youngest signers who cannot yet read.

Have conversations

Signing with your baby does not mean being silent. Actually, parents who sign find that they talk more with their child. As we discussed earlier, this talking helps your baby develop an understanding of language. Unless you are somewhere that requires silence, such as church or a wedding, *always speak with your child when you are signing*. Speak in complete sentences even though you may be using only one or two signs for the entire sentence. This will not confuse your baby. If you say, "Do you want some **MILK**?" you will only sign **MILK** for the entire sentence you are speaking.

Whenever you sign and speak, talk directly to your child. Speak clearly as you sign and give added vocal emphasis to the word or words you are signing so that your baby gets the connection between the word and the sign. When you ask, "Do you want some **MILK**?" you would accentuate the word "milk." It is also helpful to repeat the sign several times. This exaggerated signing allows your baby to see the sign you are making and associate it with the situation.

You can also have conversations with your baby about what you are doing. When your baby is nursing or drinking a bottle, you could have a conversation—albeit one-sided—with him that might go like this: "I bet you are enjoying your **MILK**. It is good **MILK**. You are so cute when you drink your **MILK**." This might seem funny to us as adults, but it really helps babies to hear the language and associate the words and signs with the activity they are engaged in.

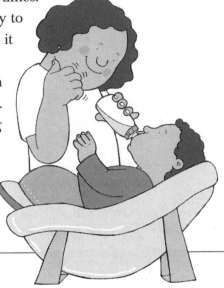

Talk and sign **MILK** when feeding your baby.

The real key to success is using the signs as often as you can in meaningful events. Every time you eat, use the **EAT** sign and use it frequently during the meal. Babies need to see things hundreds of times to learn. Say, "We're going to **EAT**. Do you want to **EAT**?" And then as you eat, say "Let's **EAT** another bite of cereal." Parents who are successful sign often. *It is less important to know a lot of signs than it is to use the signs you know.*

Engage your baby

Another important factor for success is to engage your baby in the process of signing. One of the best ways to engage your baby is to intentionally focus on him. Make the sign directly in your child's line of sight so he can see your eyes, the sign, and your mouth. Then, speak with your child, emphasizing the word you are signing. For example, you might say, "Do you want some **MORE** apple?" So many parents speak to their children with their backs turned as they are doing something else, or in the same tone they use to speak on the phone. Babies have a hard time understanding that you are speaking to them when you do these things.

You should always speak directly to your baby. Get his attention. If you are far away, come closer to him. Just the act of coming closer lets him know that you are addressing him. If he is engaged in something else, use his name and touch him to get him to look at you. Vary your tone of voice so that it is not the same tone you use to speak on the phone. If you are talking about something that has sounds associated with it, you can even make those sounds to get his attention. For example, if you are feeding him, make eating noises or say "Yummy!" If you are talking about the family dog, bark. As your baby gets older and learns more animal signs, this becomes really fun for him. He can sign **TIGER** and make a roaring sound or **ELEPHANT** and make a trumpeting sound.

> **AHA!**
>
> Learning to roll over and sit up can have an effect on your child's ability to sign. When he takes a physical or developmental leap, he may stop signing for a time. He will conquer whatever physical or developmental milestone he faces, and then you will see an increase in his ability to communicate.

Look for baby's response back

You can tell your baby is looking to you for a sign when he looks at his toy and then looks up to you, as if he is asking you for the sign. You will also know he is paying attention to your signs when he looks at your sign, then looks at his toy, and then looks back to you to see the sign again.

Often, before he can make the sign, he will respond to you with a body

AHA!

Get your whole family involved in signing. If you have older children, ask them to sign and help their younger siblings. If you see Grandma and Grandpa often, tell them what you are doing and what it will accomplish and ask them to sign. If you have another caregiver, ask her to sign with your baby. If she is hesitant, keep the number of signs small so that she does not feel overwhelmed. The more people your baby sees signing to him, the better.

smile or giggles—especially if you guess what he wants and he gets it. Sometimes he will respond even without the conscious knowledge that he is doing it. Tricia began showing Keira the **MILK** sign at four months old. Then, about one and a half months later, Keira began to make the sign. At first Tricia was unsure that what she was seeing was a sign, because Keira would squeeze her fists as she nursed. But she realized that Keira did not squeeze her hands at any other time—just when she was nursing and had been shown the **MILK** sign.

Your baby will answer you back with his looks, vocal noises, and body language before he will be able to sign or speak. Julie explains, "The first sign Isaac understood was **SLEEP.** He's six months old and if he's tired, he gets very cranky, but becomes happy as soon as he realizes we're going to put him down to sleep. Each time we put him down, we have a routine where we kiss him and then say 'Go to **SLEEP,** goodnight' then turn the light off and leave. After we leave him, he goes to sleep very quickly, so I think the sign has helped him understand what we expect of him and what we're doing each time we put him down to sleep."

Keep your eyes open—you may even see a sign this early. If not, don't be discouraged. Most babies make their first sign between seven and twelve months, because this is when they have developed the manual dexterity to sign.

Involving the family

If your baby interacts regularly with family members not in your immediate household (such as grandparents), now is a great time to introduce them to the idea of signing with your baby. Often, grandparents are amazed at the fact that they can communicate with their grandchildren at such an early age.

Pam is grandmother to Emily and several other grandchildren. She and her husband take care of four of their grandchildren daily in their home. When Pam's son and daughter-in-law decided to sign with Emily, Pam had not heard about signing with babies. She learned as Emily learned. "Emily would teach us. She signed **MILK, MORE, PLEASE, SHOES, SOCKS, COAT** and more. It was really fun and the three older cousins enjoyed it too. They learned the signs. Even though Emily is fifteen months younger than her cousins, we could understand her better. She could communicate with us." Pam says that Emily was milder and had fewer tantrums than her cousins. She talked ten months earlier than her cousins and had a larger vocabulary. "She is more confident that we know what she wants. And that is good for both of us."

ONLINE

Go to the Sign Babies website (www.signbabies. com) to see video of babies responding to signs before they can sign back! Or listen to Babies and Moms: Birth and Beyond, a radio show about signing with babies (www.babiesandmomsradio.com). Babies and Moms' website also includes videos of babies signing and lots of other great information for moms.

If you are concerned that your family members might not accept the idea of signing with your baby, check the ideas for introducing signing to caregivers in Chapter Two. Remember that your family members might be overwhelmed with the idea that they have to learn a new language (which they don't) and might resist based on their fears. Once they see a baby signing, family members often come around and embrace the idea of signing with babies.

The First Signs

As we discussed earlier, signing with your baby does not mean you are using ASL only and not speaking to him in words. You will be adding a few simple ASL signs to your regular conversations with your baby. You need to start with only a handful of signs that symbolize what you are talking about and give your baby a way to communicate back with you before he can speak.

When you start signing with your baby, concentrate on the activities you do each day and the things that you notice your baby is interested in. These are the best signs to start with, because these experiences occur often and give you opportunities to sign. Here, the activities are broken down into categories to help you group them together. Don't worry about having to learn a lot of signs. Just learn the few signs for each activity and go from there.

As your baby grows, add signs for each activity. This way you don't have to feel overwhelmed that you have to remember a lot of signs at once. If you have a hard time remembering the signs to use while changing diapers, copy the diaper/ dressing signs and post them next to the diaper changing station. Place the meal signs next to the high chair and so forth. This way, you will have a reference on display right where you need it and you won't have to rummage through an alphabetized dictionary to find the sign you need. Part II includes suggested signs for each activity.

TWO CENTS

If you are the type of person who likes learning from a teacher, consider taking a baby sign language class. There are instructors across the country that teach classes and can help you learn the signs. Just make sure that the instructor you choose teaches ASL signs. There is no need to learn "baby signs" suggested by some instructors, because all babies can sign ASL signs. A great place to start looking for instructors is the Sign Babies website (www.signbabies.com) or the Sign2Me Classes (www.sign2me. com/classes.php).

Meal signs

MILK

Eating is one of the best times to sign with your baby. If you are starting to sign at four months, you will be limited mostly to making the sign for **MILK**. You can use this sign for nursing or bottle-feeding. Parents get hung up on the delivery mechanism–breast or bottle–but babies don't have an issue. It is milk to them. If you are worried that there may be some confusion about this, rest assured that thousands of nursing moms have used the sign **MILK** for nursing and their babies have not been confused. When you anticipate that your baby is hungry, ask him "Do you want some **MILK**? Are you ready for some **MILK**?"

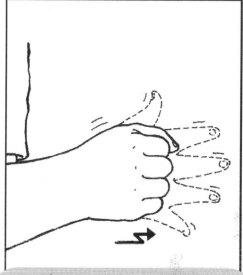

Note: This sign is also used for nursing or for milk in a bottle.

If you can nurse or feed a bottle one-handed, go ahead and have a conversation with your baby while you are feeding him. "Yum. This **MILK** is so good. You are so cute when you drink your **MILK**." And so forth. Don't worry about looking silly. This is a time for you to look into your baby's eyes and talk and sign with him. It really helps. Just don't "converse" with your baby in the middle of the night. Sleep is too precious, and your baby needs to learn that nighttime feedings are not a time for conversations, or else he may wake up and look for your company even when he is not hungry.

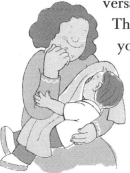

Sign **MILK** while nursing.

Be careful of using certain signs out of context. If you are ready to feed your baby, then make the sign for **MILK** and tell your baby you are ready. If you sign **MILK** out of context, you might make him unhappy. For example, if you are talking to a friend about how your baby can respond to **MILK**, but you are not ready to feed him, he might become angry when he sees the sign but the milk doesn't follow. He has come to expect that when he hears you talking about milk and signing it, he is going to eat.

Ruby had to nurse whenever we discussed and signed **MILK** in a class I taught. It became a joke in our class, but was not so funny for her mom. **MILK** is a sign for a specific thing for your baby—eating. Use it when you want to feed him. There are some other signs such as **MORE** that can be used in many situations without trouble. We will discuss this later.

ALL DONE/FINISHED

This helps signify that the feeding activity is over. **ALL DONE** is a great sign to use at other times. When you want your baby to understand that you are finished doing one thing and are moving on to another, this sign is very useful. You can tell him that his bath is **ALL DONE,** or that you are **FINISHED** reading the book.

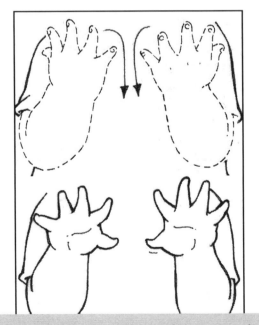

ALL DONE: Show that there is nothing in your hand

MORE

As your baby matures, you will want to add the sign **MORE.** **MORE** is a magical sign for babies. It gives them the power to get **MORE** of what they want. When you are feeding your baby, they can ask for **MORE** apples, **MORE** banana, **MORE** of everything. This is a powerful tool for babies, who seem to want **MORE** of everything.

When you are feeding your baby, you can introduce **MORE** by feeding your baby a few bites of rice cereal or banana and then asking him, "Would you like some **MORE**?" Make the sign

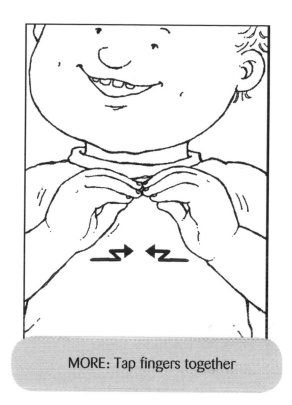

MORE: Tap fingers together

and then pick up the spoon and feed him more. As your interactions become more complex, you can even add two signs together and ask her, "Do you want **MORE** to **EAT**?" Eventually, as your child grows, these sign pairs will grow as well.

EAT

As you progress to solid foods, use the sign **EAT** to introduce your baby to eating. At first, it is not necessary to show the signs for different foods. Signing **EAT** helps your baby understand that the activity of eating will occur. Just as with the **MILK** sign, have a conversation. "Are you hungry? Do you want to **EAT**? Let's get you some **FOOD**." Luckily **FOOD** and **EAT** are the same sign. Continue your conversation as you feed your baby.

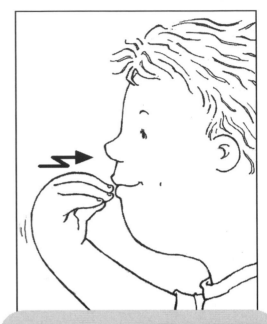

EAT: Like putting food in your mouth

AHA!

Use the hand you write with—your dominant hand—for all one-handed signs like **EAT** and for finger spelling. If you switch hands while signing, it is no big deal. But a deaf person would consider that something like a stutter, because it momentarily confuses the rhythm of an ASL conversation. Sign correctly now so you don't "stutter" if you ever decide to learn ASL. When a sign requires both hands, your dominant hand will be the hand that moves and your other hand will act as a base. When both hands move at the same time, the hand shapes are almost always the same.

AHA!

If you don't know the sign for something, don't stress out. You can use a generic sign for an entire category of things. For example, use the sign **EAT** or **FOOD** for the process of eating and for the foods. Later, you can learn the signs for specific foods such as banana, apple, cookie, cracker and so forth.

YES

When you ask your child to respond to a request such as "Do you want more **BANANA**?" your child may be able to sign **YES** more easily than sign **BANANA**. **YES** works well because your baby can sign it to say yes to a specific type of food. However, because you might not want to give your child choices at this early age, you can introduce **YES** now and then reinforce it once you are giving your child more choices in food selection—generally starting some time between eight and twelve months.

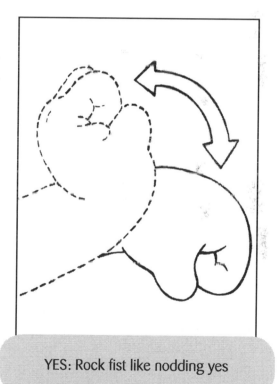

YES: Rock fist like nodding yes

Diaper/Dressing signs

CHANGE

Because you are changing diapers six to ten times a day, it's great to have a way to let your baby know that you are going to change his diaper. The sign **CHANGE** is especially useful for babies who do not like to stop and lie still. Often, when babies learn that **CHANGE** means only a momentary stop in their play, they will relax and allow their parents to change their diapers. Right now, your four-month old might passively lie on the changing table and let you change his diaper, but just think how it will be when he's mobile and wants to go, go, go!

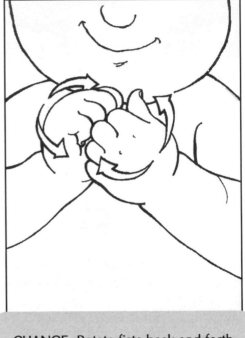

CHANGE: Rotate fists back and forth

Don't be surprised later–when your baby is walking–if he comes to you and lets you know that he needs his diaper changed. This is a common occurrence among parents who sign with their babies. Even before the tell-tale smell appears, babies often tell their parents that they need a change. Starting with **CHANGE** now can also help you later when it's time to potty train because your baby has been aware of his bodily functions and has a way to explain them much earlier–another plus to look forward to.

CLOTHES/GET DRESSED

The sign for **CLOTHES** is also the sign for the entire phrase **GET DRESSED** or **PUT ON CLOTHES**. Tell your baby, "We are going to **GET DRESSED**. You have such beautiful **CLOTHES**." Then, as you dress your baby, explain the names of each piece of clothing. Later, you can learn the signs for these as well. Telling your baby the names of each clothing item helps increase his vocabulary and it gives you something to talk about while dressing him. Later, this becomes useful when you need to put on shoes and socks before going out and your fourteen-month old is resisting.

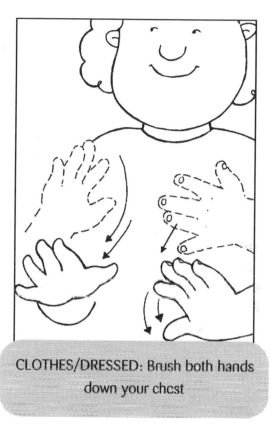

CLOTHES/DRESSED: Brush both hands down your chest

LIGHT or FAN

Babies spend a lot of time on their backs looking up at the lights. Because your baby is on his back when you are dressing him, **LIGHT** can be a useful distraction sign. If your baby notices the lights, comment on them and say, "Yes, you are looking at the **LIGHT**. It is bright." For the same reason that **LIGHT** is a great sign to know during dressing time, **FAN** works well too, if there is a fan where you dress your baby.

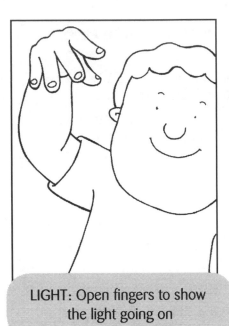

LIGHT: Open fingers to show the light going on

If you have a freestanding fan, you might want to introduce this sign later. When my son was about fourteen months old, he was looking at his fan in his room and he signed **FAN** and **AIRPLANE** and pointed to the fan as well. It took me a moment to realize what he was saying, but I soon understood that he was commenting that the **FAN** was shaped like the propeller on his **AIRPLANE** that we had been playing with just a few minutes earlier. He was making associations at such a young age.

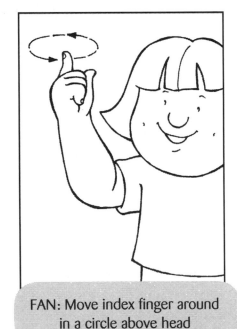

FAN: Move index finger around in a circle above head

AHA!

A great bonus to signing with your baby is that you can explain why he should not do something, instead of just saying "No." For example, FAN will be useful later in conjunction with HURT or NO TOUCH. You can teach your baby that the FAN will HURT his finger if he touches it. When you explain that the reason he can't touch something is that it can HURT him, your child is more apt to listen.

ALL DONE/FINISHED

ALL DONE is helpful when diapering because it helps give your baby a sense that this activity is complete. Some babies do not like to be diapered and when they know that they will be told the activity is over, it can help them endure the process. Even the happiest baby likes to know what is going on in his world. **ALL DONE** helps you accomplish this.

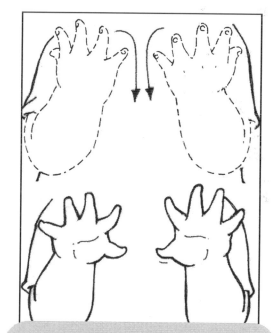

ALL DONE: Show that there is nothing in your hand

UP

UP is the simplest sign of all—you just point up. By pointing up and saying "Let's get **UP**?" when a diaper change is done, you give him a signal for what is going to happen next. With time, he will let you know that he wants **UP** from his high chair, car seat, or the bed. This sign can also be used to say **PICK ME UP**.

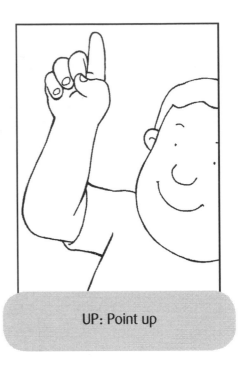

UP: Point up

MASSAGE

Baby massage can calm children, help them with colic, help their digestion, help them to sleep longer and give both of you a feeling of bonding. When my son was a baby, we usually massaged him before getting dressed for bed. We spent five to ten minutes giving him a massage and helping him to relax. It got to the point that when we would say, "Let's have a **MASSAGE**," you could see his body begin to relax on its own. Actually, one of his first words was "massage," but he just said "sage."

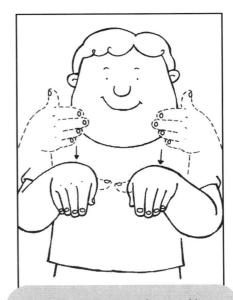

MASSAGE: Move fingers like massaging shoulders

Activity signs
BOOK

The American Academy of Pediatrics suggests that you read with your baby for fifteen to twenty minutes a day. Reading introduces your baby to language and sounds that help him develop his linguistic abilities. Some parents also report that daily reading gives their child a time to slow down during the day. Before you pick up a book and begin to read, say to your baby, "We are going to read a **BOOK**. Let's choose a **BOOK** to read."

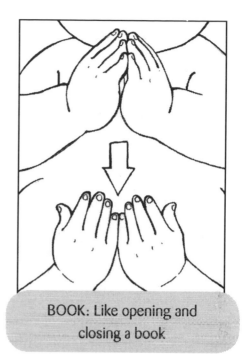

BOOK: Like opening and closing a book

ALL DONE/FINISHED

ALL DONE is helpful when you want to transition from one playtime activity to another. Think about it from a baby's perspective. He is having a great time dropping the ball off the highchair and watching you pick it up (he is learning about gravity and cause and effect). But you get tired. **ALL DONE** can help you explain to your child that you are finished picking up the ball and are going to move on to another activity.

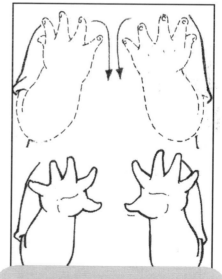

ALL DONE: Show that there is nothing in your hand

PLAY

When your baby is four months old, you might not be playing a lot with him in the way you commonly think about play. But you can use the sign **PLAY** for the times when you are doing tummy time and interacting on the floor. Then, as your baby gets older and is playing more, the sign helps him to indicate that he wants to play with you. By signing now, you can help prepare your baby for playtime and tummy time.

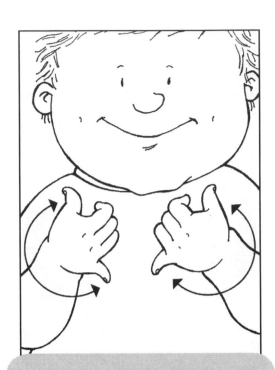

PLAY: Index and pinkie stick out and hands swing back and forth

Most babies cannot correctly make the sign for play until they are well over twelve months because they do not have the manual dexterity needed to lift only the thumb and pinkie. That, however, won't stop your baby from making the sign to the best of his ability. Generally, babies will make this sign some time around ten to fourteen months old, but it may look more like shaking fists or open hands.

MUSIC/SING/SONG

Babies love music. As your baby grows, introduce him to music through children's CDs, lullaby CDs, your favorite music, and even your singing. Watch how his face lights up when he hears music. Teaching him the sign for **MUSIC** later gives him the ability to request music or comment on the music he is listening to. Throughout the book and in Appendix C, specific songs that are great to sign with your baby are recommended. Music is one of my eleven-year-old daughter Anna's favorite signs.

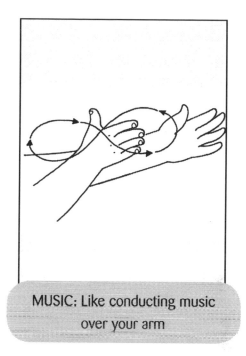

MUSIC: Like conducting music over your arm

CAR

Your baby may spend a lot of time in the car or seeing cars drive by. **CAR** can help your baby understand that you are going to drive in the car. It also makes a great sign for playtime when you have toy cars that your baby plays with. Babies do not need to know the specific signs for truck, bus, and car at this age—for the most part they are generalists and don't need the specifics. But, if your child gets really interested in transportation or in construction, you might find yourself learning the specific signs for different modes of transportation and construction.

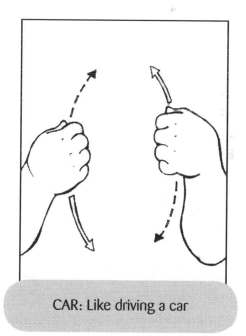

CAR: Like driving a car

DOG or CAT

If you have a family pet, the sign for **DOG** or **CAT** can be very useful. Also, if you frequently visit a park where people bring their dogs, this sign will be one that you will want to use. Babies are very interested in animals and often their first animal contact is with a dog or a cat.

You can also use this sign when reading books that include stories about dogs or cats. You can comment on dogs or cats that you see on the street or at a friend's house. Later, when your baby wants to pet the dog, you can use this sign to teach him to **PET** the **DOG SOFT**.

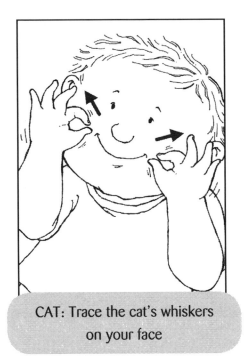

CAT: Trace the cat's whiskers on your face

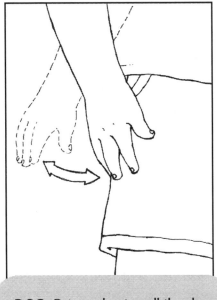

DOG: Pat you leg to call the dog

BEAR

Your baby may have a special friend such as a teddy bear that he plays with or sleeps with. At this young age, the bear may not have great significance but later the bear may become a *transitional object*— an object that helps your baby in times when he transitions from being with you to being with a caregiver or going to sleep alone. If you also incorporate the bear into your play, learn the sign **BEAR** to signify the importance of your baby's "friend" in your together play.

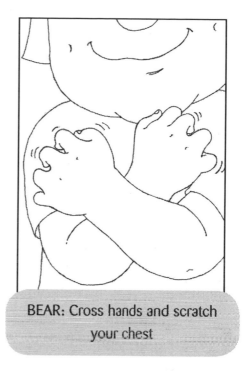

BEAR: Cross hands and scratch your chest

BABY

Babies love to know that they are the baby. At this age, your baby will not recognize himself as separate from you. This comes at a later age. However, you can ask him "Who is that **BABY**?" when you show him a mirror and he sees herself. This is an especially fun game to play with babies around six months and beyond. Later, your baby will recognize his place in the family. I remember the day when my son came and signed to me "I'm the **BABY**" by pointing to himself and signing **BABY**. He knew his place in the world and was very pleased to understand that.

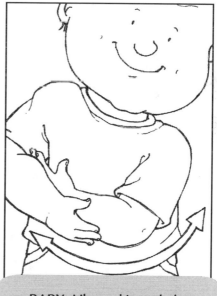

BABY: Like rocking a baby

MORE

Babies want more of the things they enjoy. You can use **MORE** when you play with your baby to help him ask you for more of what he wants to play. Ask him, "Do you want **MORE** tickling?" Anything you play together, you can ask if he wants **MORE**. If you toss your baby in the air or blow raspberries on his tummy or tickle his toes, he will soon learn to sign **MORE** to keep you going!

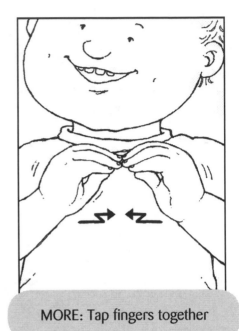

MORE: Tap fingers together

YES

As was discussed with mealtime signs, **YES** works well when you want to give your baby a choice. If you see that your child can choose between two activities, introduce **YES**. If you still need to lead activities, save **YES** for a later time when he can make choices.

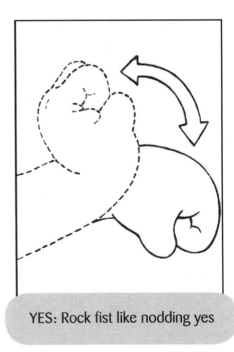

YES: Rock fist like nodding yes

Bath signs
BATH

To help your baby transition to bathing, tell him "We are going to give you a **BATH**." The sign for **BATH** is great to start with at four months. It helps prepare your baby for his bath and gets him in the right frame of mind. Do not worry about making the sign **BATH** *during* the bath at this young age. You need to keep both hands on your baby. As he grows and can sit up on his own, then you can comment about the bath.

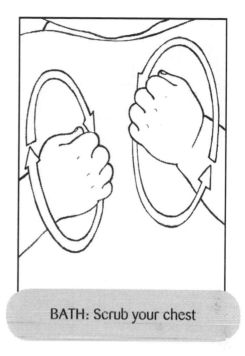

BATH: Scrub your chest

ALL DONE/FINISHED

When you are ready to take your baby from the bath, let him know this. Say, "We are **ALL DONE** with your bath. Let's get out now." If your baby loves the water and throws a fit when the bath is done, this should help ease the transition. Again, never make a sign if you need to have both hands on your baby to maintain a safe bathing experience. If you need to wait, tell him when you are drying him that the bath is all done and discuss this with him then. You could say, "Our bath is **ALL DONE**. Now we need to get dry and **GET DRESSED**."

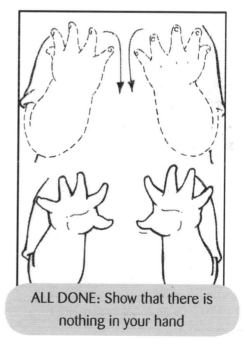

ALL DONE: Show that there is nothing in your hand

Bedtime signs

BOOK

If story time is a part of the bedtime ritual, sign **BOOK** and let
your baby know that you are
going to read a bedtime story.
One of the books that we love in
our family is Sandra Boynton's
Going to Bed Book. We have read
this so often in our house that
everyone can quote it by memory,
including our son who now says it
to his sister. Make sure you sign
BOOK before you sign **SLEEP**
or **BED**, so that your baby does
not get confused as to the order of
your ritual.

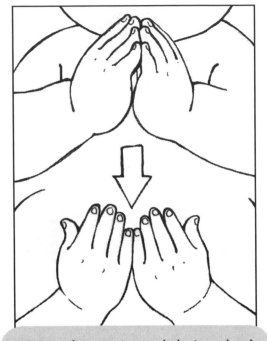

BOOK: Like opening and closing a book

SLEEP or BED

Babies need help transitioning to sleep. If you start signing **SLEEP** or **BED** now, when you get him ready for bed and put him to bed, then he will begin to understand this process, and will eventually even be able to tell you when he needs to go to sleep. Because babies have no way to communicate, they cry when they are tired and want to sleep. Babies who sign can tell their parents they are tired and some babies will do that.

My son came to me during our playtime and looked and me and signed **SLEEP**. He was tired of playing and ready for bed. After that, he often let me know he was ready for **SLEEP** and napping became a joyful part of the day for both of us. Start using this sign now and it will pay big dividends in the near future.

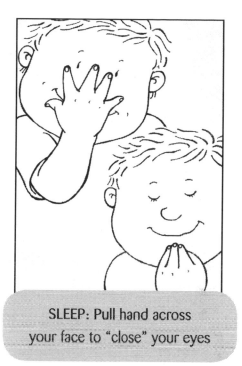

SLEEP: Pull hand across your face to "close" your eyes

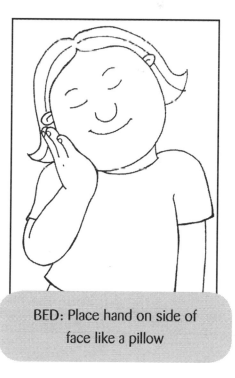

BED: Place hand on side of face like a pillow

MUSIC/SING/SONG

Experts highly recommend that you include a song in your bedtime ritual to quiet your baby and prepare him for sleep. If you sing a nightly lullaby, let your baby know that it is time. "We are going to **SING** our favorite lullaby. You can choose a song that you can sign, or learn signs to a song that you love. Don't worry if you don't have a great voice. Your baby loves to hear you sing and this time is a wonderful time to create bonds.

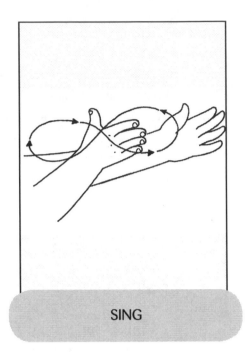

SING

BEAR

Your baby may have a special friend such as a teddy bear that he sleeps with to help him transition from being with you to going to sleep alone. Learn the sign **BEAR** so that your baby will have a way to signify this important transitional object later when he needs it. If your baby has a blanket or a bunny or a doll, the sign for these words are in Part II.

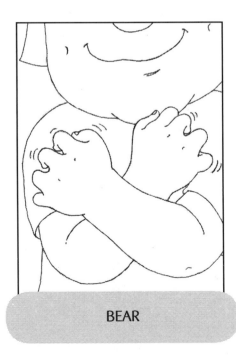

BEAR

A Final Note on Incorporating Sign into Life

Incorporate signing into your life and make it an activity that isn't separate from your regular interactions with your baby. You might feel a bit strange having conversations with your baby before he can speak, but it is very important to do this and you will soon find it enjoyable. You can incorporate signing into your reading time, for example. Say and sign to him that you are going to read a book and then sign whatever pictures you know the signs for. Go beyond just reading the story. Even the simple act of labeling the pictures in the story—telling what each object on the page is while pointing to it—helps to develop your baby's linguistic abilities.

Summary

In this chapter, we discussed:

☆ How your baby is developing from four to seven months

☆ How to start signing with your baby

☆ What signs to start signing with your baby

Bottom Line

Now is the time to start signing with your baby. Begin with just a few signs and then add more signs as your baby begins doing new things, such as playing and eating.

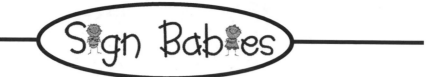

Chapter Four

Eight to Twelve Months— Watch Me Sign

For most babies, the period from eight to twelve months is a time when they get mobile. Imagine what that must feel like. Finally a chance to get where you want to go! Even though you may not be ready, your decorating will probably go from Grown Up Chic to Child Proof Sensible, with everything you love placed higher than 2 feet off the floor, cabinets and dressers secured to the wall, locks installed on the toilets and cabinets, and outlet covers everywhere.

This is also the time when most babies make their first sign—even if you have been signing with them from birth. They now have the motor development to make signs, and if you have been signing with them for a few weeks or months, they have been primed for sign!

In this chapter, we'll take a look at the following:
☆ How your baby is developing from eight to twelve months
☆ What to expect from your baby's first signing attempts
☆ Strategies to increase your child's ability to sign
☆ Common questions and problems parents encounter
☆ Signs and activities to use in this period

JUST BEGINNING NOW? If you haven't started signing with your baby yet, it's okay. You have not missed the window of opportunity. Go back and read Chapter Three: 4 to 7 Months–I'm Ready to Start to get the basics of how to sign with your baby. Then continue with this chapter.

Your Baby's Development

Your baby is probably a ball of constant motion–with so many new things to learn and do, it is no wonder she doesn't want to sit still. She is exploring her newfound ability to sit up by herself, her ability to pick up things and examine them, and her ability to crawl or scoot on her bottom. She is now standing while holding onto the couch. She might even be ready to walk with the assistance of a table or couch. If she is really ready to move, she may be walking by the end of this period with little assistance.

Motor development

While standing is a great milestone, your baby is also making great accomplishments in other areas of physical development that will aid her ability to sign. She is now learning to grasp objects with the pincer grasp–using her thumb and first or second finger. This means that your baby can make a wider variety of signs that were not physically possible for her before.

The pincer grasp

She is also learning to bang things together, another useful skill for signing words such as **MORE** and **BALL**. Toward the end of this period, she will also have mastered the skill of taking things out of a container, a move that takes great spatial acuity and coordination. She will begin to poke with her index finger and may even try to imitate writing or scribbling.

Many parents notice that their baby signs **MORE** by poking her index finger on the palm of her hand. This is a very common adaptation of the sign for **MORE** and is often made during this time when babies are still developing the ability to manipulate their index finger. You should keep signing **MORE** correctly and your baby will adapt over time. Don't worry about correcting her sign, unless your baby is very receptive to your showing her how to sign it correctly. If you continue to sign it correctly while still responding to her modification, she will change it over time on her own.

You may also notice that one of her hands seems more developed in terms of motor skills than the other. Not to worry, as babies will sometimes prefer one hand over the other. This does not necessarily mean that if she prefers the left hand, she will be left-handed. The identification of her dominant hand comes much later.

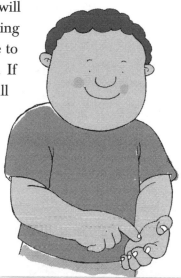

Some babies sign **MORE** by pointing an index finger on the palm of the other hand.

Language development

Most babies whose parents have signed with them since four to seven months will sign during this time. According to the American Academy of Pediatrics, even babies whose parents have not signed with them will now begin to point and gesture for things they want. Because you have been signing with your baby, her abilities will now begin to blossom and you may even see an explosion of signs. Hearing babies of deaf parents typically sign between fifty and one hundred signs by their first birthday. Don't worry if you think you can't remember that many signs. You don't need to learn them all at the same time, and if you use only ten to twenty signs, your relationship with your baby will still be easier than if you didn't sign at all.

Your baby will also increase her verbal communications with you. Her earlier coos and gurgles will turn into more recognizable syllables such as "ba," "da," "ga," and "ma." She may even say words such as "bye-bye" or "mama." You can use these experiences to reinforce language learning. For the most

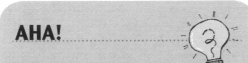

AHA!

Babies who are born deaf or hearing impaired babble, but they babble with their fingers. Some mothers of hearing babies who sign with their babies also report that their babies babble with their fingers and with their voices as well. This is an interesting glimpse into the way language develops, and shows that babble is an important stage in language learning—whether you can speak or not.

part, her first syllables are not requests for something—rather she is practicing the sounds. You can, however, turn these first utterances into meaningful expressions by giving them meaning. For example, if your baby says "ma ma ma ma," say and sign to her, "Oh, it sounds like you are saying **MAMA**. I am your **MAMA**. Can you say **MAMA**?" You are teaching her that her random noises can also mean words. Sign as you teach her so that she knows the sign associated with that sound as well.

But not everything is random for your baby at this age. She now understands many of the words you have been saying and signing to her for months. She knows her name and she can now understand when you sign and ask her questions such as "Do you want some **MILK**?" She may express her understanding with squeals or grunts or flailing arms, or she may even make the **MILK** sign back to you as a way of saying, "Yes, I do want some **MILK**." She may become excited when you ask whether she wants to take a bath and sign **BATH**. She probably understands more words and signs than you think.

One of the very most effective things you can do to increase your baby's linguistic comprehension is to speak with her as much as possible. Talking with your baby is one of the best ways to help her learn the linguistic game. Have simple conversations with her

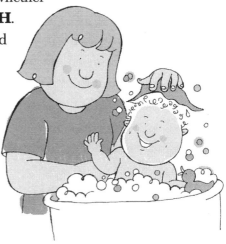

about what you are doing: "We are taking a **BATH**. Don't you love taking a **BATH**? I love the **WATER**. It feels so good to have your toes **WASHED**." If she can see you and your hands are free and *it is safe to sign*, sign with her at the same time you talk to her. You don't need to sign everything in the sentence. Just sign one or two signs in each sentence.

If you speak another language in the home (in addition to the signing you are doing), you might be concerned that your baby will be confused by hearing both

languages. Research shows that when children are exposed to two or more languages (this includes signing) at the earliest ages, they are able to learn both languages simultaneously—especially if they are both spoken consistently. Your baby will probably become more proficient in the dominant home language and she may interject words from one language into the other. But in time, she will learn to distinguish the two languages. Using sign language can help your baby learn both spoken languages better. Use the same signs while speaking both languages. For example, sign **MILK** whether you are saying "milk" in English or your spouse is saying "leche" in Spanish.

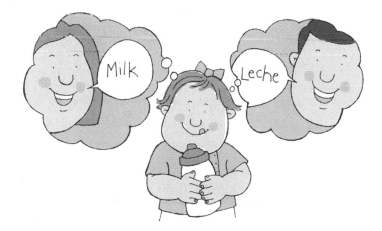

Being bilingual or trilingual is an incredible gift to give your child. Start speaking both languages in the home as soon as you can. If one parent is fluent in only one language, have that parent speak that language and let the parent who is bilingual speak the other language. If grandparents or other caregivers who spend significant amounts of time with your baby speak another language, encourage them to do so around her. Teach them the same signs to use in both languages. The earlier you start your child and the more exposure she has, the more capable she will be at both languages. She will not be hindered in school. Research actually suggests that children who learn two or more languages (signing counts as a second language in this research) have better abilities in both languages and show an increase in IQ.

Cognitive development

At eight months, your baby is curious about everything around her. She does, however, have a short attention span. Don't take it personally if you can't get through *Good Night Moon* without her mind wandering. Her attention span is actually about two to three minutes. By twelve months, your baby may be more willing to sit for ten to fifteen minutes if some object is particularly interesting, but don't count on it. She will generally be a ball of motion most of the time. This is one reason not to "teach" signs. "Teaching" conjures up images of sitting still for long periods of time, actively trying to learn. Instead, incorporate signing in to everything you do. This chapter includes great activities that incorporate cognitive learning and signing.

Your baby is also very interested in the details of things and interactions now. She can spend time looking at objects, feeling textures, and experimenting to discover the consequences of her actions. This is the time when she will want to drop things off her high chair repeatedly to see what happens. You are part of her experiment. She will watch you intently to see what you do. This is one reason why most babies begin to sign in this period.

As she explores and experiments, she can become frustrated. Don't jump in too soon. Let your baby learn to handle small frustrations now so that she can handle greater frustrations in the future. Be available for her when she becomes too confused or upset, but stand back a bit and let her learn. Sometimes the most golden learning moments come when she is a bit frustrated and works the situation out on her own.

Social development

This period is also a time for separation anxiety. Your baby may have easily gone to others before, but now she only wants you. This may even occur with the people she is around frequently, such as grandparents or caregivers. Your baby is reaching one of the first emotional milestones in her life. She is realizing that there is only one you—the first love of her life. She can now distinguish you from others, and she associates you with her well-being.

Even though this stage generally passes quickly, it can be stressful for both you and your child. Separation anxiety also occurs because your baby now understands *object permanence*—the idea that something or someone still exists when your baby cannot see it or them. Don't be surprised if your baby soon begins to cry if you leave the room, as she now knows that you exist somewhere she is not. Generally, this reaction occurs sometime between the fifth and sixth month and intensifies through the tenth month.

Socially, your baby now has to learn about rules and limits. Because this is a time of new mobility, your baby is bound to get into things she shouldn't. She might need to learn not to touch certain objects at a relative's house, or how to interact with the family dog. Often, distracting her is the best method to quickly solve the situation. If she is heading for the Ming vase, distract her and turn her attention toward the cuddly bear you are holding by changing your tone of voice to get her attention. Say something such as, "Look at this wonderful **BEAR**. Doesn't this **BEAR** look like fun to play with?" This often works better than using the word "no"

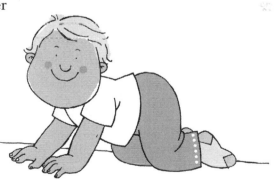

and expecting her to react. Her emotions and thought processes may not allow her to stop doing what she is headed for.

However, learning not to do something she really wants to do is a major step toward learning self-control, and there will be times when she needs to know that something or someone is off limits. Babies who sign may have an easier time with limits, because they have a way to express these limits. Teaching your baby the signs for **STOP, NO TOUCH, SOFT TOUCH, LOOK, WAIT,** and **HELP** will give her a way to understand what you expect of her. Keep your rules simple and stay consistent. This is the best way to teach your child how to react in each situation. But do not expect too much and be very patient and loving. Your baby is still developing and has very little sense of self-control.

AHA!

The parent who signs and explains why a child should or should not do things may find that as the child matures, she is capable of very intense understanding and has advanced skills of negotiation. This is a double-edged sword. You can explain to your baby why something should not be done or how something needs to happen and skip tantrums. But her advanced understanding helps her negotiate with you at a very early age—sometime around eighteen to twenty-four months.

Respond to the things your baby does well. This is as important and effective as teaching babies self-control. If your baby hesitates, as if to ask for permission before touching something that is questionable, let her know that you noticed and value this response. This reinforces good behavior. You can say, "**THANK YOU** for asking before you took the doll. It makes me so **HAPPY**." You will increasingly have opportunities to use positive reinforcement as your baby matures. By saying **THANK YOU**, you are modeling good manners and introducing the concept of good manners that your baby will learn later on.

Now the Signing Fun Begins

It's a wonderful time for signing, as your baby works out the communication game. She will begin to understand the connection between what she does with her hands and how you respond to her. That is why your baby will probably sign back to you—especially if you have been signing with her for a few months. Babies have the manual dexterity to make signs now, and they have the cognitive and social development to want to communicate their needs. When signing "clicks" with her, she will pick up signs more quickly. She may even begin to sign several different signs at once.

At times, it may even seem that she is bursting with desire to communicate. She will look at you for the name and sign for everything she sees. Depending on how many signs you introduce to your baby, your baby will be able to recognize twenty to one hundred signs by her first birthday. She will make some of these signs, and some she may not be able to make yet. There are some signs that babies may never make. What busy baby that is on the move wants to make the sign for **"WAIT"**? She may understand the concept and the sign when you make it, but she probably won't sign it back.

In addition to the signs she is learning, your baby may even have a vocabulary of two to four spoken words to go along with her signs—even if you are the only one who can understand her when she says them. If she doesn't say anything comprehensible, don't worry. Gibberish is good, too.

TWO CENTS

Many parents and caregivers feel overwhelmed by the idea of learning dozens of signs. If you feel overwhelmed, just remember that you don't need to learn all the signs at once. You need to learn only a few signs at a time for each activity. Even five signs make a big difference. Before you know it, you will have learned dozens of signs. If you have a caregiver who is overwhelmed, copy out five signs from this book or give the caregiver the five signs from the *Sign Babies ASL Flash Cards* and ask him or her to start with these signs.

Introducing signs for things baby sees

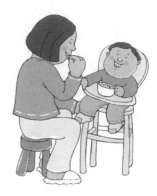

At this age, your baby understands that things have specific names. She will look to you to show her the names of everything in her world. This action is called *labeling*. Have you seen that look when she sees something and then stares at you as if to ask, "What is that, Mom?"

Tell her what things are called, and if you know the sign for that thing, sign it too. It is important to use the actual words for things and not made-up words. This increases your baby's vocabulary and helps her gain a better grasp on the language. Although it is cute to say "Do you want a ba ba?" your baby is better served by hearing the word "bottle" and seeing the sign. The same is true for words that your baby will begin to approximate in speech. If your baby says "ba ba" for her bottle, use the word "bottle" instead of repeating "ba ba," so that she hears and learns the correct word.

Because your baby wants to know the names of things and their signs, this becomes a great time to new signs for the things around you. If you have not learned signs for your child's favorite toys or foods, now is a good time. Animal signs are also very useful to know because children love animals and baby books have lots of animals in them.

Make sure that you ask your baby questions about what she is looking at so that she can use her ability and learn more names. For example, when you are reading a book, say and sign, "See the **BIRD**? Can you show me the **BIRD**?" She may be able point to it in the book and make the sign for it. This type of recognition shows that she knows the names and the signs for objects, and it will strengthen as she gets closer to her first birthday. If your baby is receptive when she is eight months old, take her hand and point it at the pictures in the book as you talk about them.

IMPORTANT: Many parents ask about is how to sign a person's name. Specific name signs are given only by people in the deaf community. Hearing people should not create their own name signs because the sign could stand for something else—possibly something offensive. You can use a generic sign such as **MOM, DAD,** or **GRANDMA**. When you need to differentiate between people or animals, use a name indicator. Sign the first letter of the person's name over the heart. This is like calling someone by his initials. If you have more than one person with the same first letter, try a combination of both letters, or sign the first letter next to the head for a male or next to the jaw for a female.

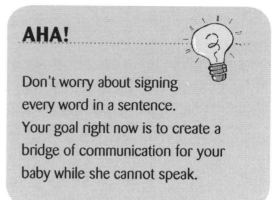

AHA!

Don't worry about signing every word in a sentence. Your goal right now is to create a bridge of communication for your baby while she cannot speak.

Increasing baby's signing abilities

There are several things you can do to help increase your baby's signing abilities. There are some basic things you should always do and some additional things you can do if the situation is right. Always do the following:

☆ Make sure that you get your baby's attention before you sign to her. Babies at this age are busy and on the move. Call her name, change your tone of voice, or touch your baby to get her attention.

☆ Make sure that you sign directly in your baby's line of sight. Make sure she can see your face and hands at the same time. This helps your baby to see your mouth, hear your voice, and see the sign (see the illustration.)

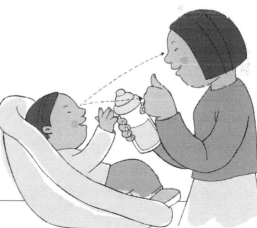

☆ Make sure you and your baby are looking at the same thing. If she is looking at the bird and you are looking at the dog, she might get confused when you show her the sign for **DOG**.

In addition to getting your baby's attention and signing in front of your baby, you can also try the following techniques:

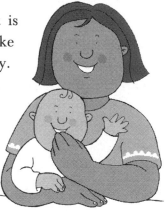

☆ Sign on your baby's body. Sometimes, it is effective to get behind your baby and make the sign on her body or in front of her body. This helps your baby see what the sign looks like from the signer's perspective. For example, hold your baby on your lap and sign **EAT** right on her mouth (see the illustration).

☆ Help your baby make the sign. If your baby is receptive to having her hands manipulated, you can help her form the signs. Some children don't like to have their hands formed, so if your baby doesn't like this, don't worry.

☆ Point to the object you are signing. If your baby can see the object that you are signing, point to the object so your baby will know what you are signing. This is especially effective when you are reading books and signing or when you are pointing out objects in your house such as food or toys.

By far, the most important key to increasing your baby's signing ability is to sign the signs you have chosen in as many situations as you can and as regularly as you can. If you are going to sign only five signs, use these signs often and in different situations. This will lead to more success than signing dozens of signs sporadically.

Sign as you read

Reading to babies is a great way to encourage language development on several levels. When you read out loud, you introduce your child to the rich sound of language. You also introduce her to the concept of words on a page. When you add signing to your reading experience, you make this process an interactive experience. Babies not only see the words and pictures and hear the sounds, but they also participate by signing along with you. Reading books becomes a fun and interesting experience for everyone.

> **AHA!**
>
> ASL does not have the same syntax or structure as English sentences, and sometimes one sign stands for a complete thought. For example, the sign **COAT** also means "Put on your coat."

Reading reinforces the concept that everything has a name and a sign (called *labeling*). Say, "Let's read a **BOOK**. Which **BOOK** should we read tonight?" Choose books with simple stories and pictures of things relevant to your baby. Board books or cloth books are great because they allow your baby to interact with the book by turning the pages. Books with simple but colorful illustrations are best.

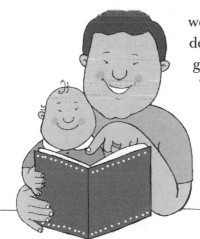

Choose your favorite books and sign any of the words you know. If you can't sign the entire book, don't worry. You can always learn more signs. A great book to start with is *Brown Bear, Brown Bear*. This book is very repetitive and helps you sign a lot of animal signs. Another option is to put the *Sign Babies ASL Flash Cards* for the signs you are signing in a 4 x 6 photo album and make your own personal "book" that you know includes the signs you want to use with your baby.

Note: Throughout Baby Signing 1-2-3, there are suggestions for great books to read and sign with your baby. There is also a comprehensive list of books and their topics in Appendix C.

Books become even more important in your baby's world as they give her an opportunity to show you what she knows. Take a step back and let your baby lead the reading process. If she knows a few signs, let her express her knowledge by signing things she sees in the book. You can ask her questions about what she sees in the book and ask her to show you things in the book. If she signs something, reinforce the sign with the spoken word for that sign: "Yes, that is a **BIRD**!"

How to read and sign

When you read and sign, you will wish you were an octopus. Two hands can't sign and hold a book *and* keep track of a wiggly baby. Don't worry. You can do it with a bit of practice and adaptation. Here are a few suggestions to try:

☆ If you and your spouse are reading with your baby together, ask your spouse to hold the book while you read and sign. This has the added dimension of showing your baby that reading is important to both parents. Switch and have your spouse read and sign so that your baby has the chance to hear both voices read.

☆ If you are alone with your baby, put her on your lap and find a pillow to prop the book up. Then sign between the book and your baby's gaze (see illustration.)

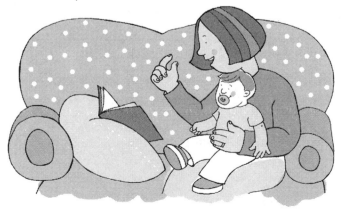

✩ You can also hold the book with one hand and sign signs with the other hand. If you are reading an animal book while holding your baby, you can sign the animal signs on her body such as **ELEPHANT, GIRAFFE,** and so forth. Babies get a kick out of this and it usually results in lots of giggles. If signs are made with two hands, use your baby as the "second hand," signing the signs on her body. For example, if you need to sign **BEAR**, tap one side of the **BEAR** sign on your baby's hand (see illustration.)

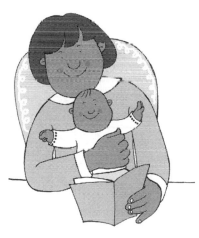

TWO CENTS

Here is a list of some of our favorite books and the signs you can do with them:

Very Hungry Caterpillar by Eric Carle: food signs

Moo, Baa La La La! by Sandra Boynton: animal signs

Brown Bear, Brown Bear by Eric Carle: animal signs

The Going to Bed Book by Sandra Boynton: bedtime and bath time signs

Curious George Are You Curious? by H.A. Rey: signs for emotions

Hug by Jez Alborough: signs for emotions

Counting Kisses by Karen Katz: signs for family members

Blue Hat, Green Hat by Sandra Boynton: colors

Don't stress out and get too worried about signing everything. Do what you can. Soon, you will be reading and your baby will be signing, so you won't need to be such an octopus.

Sign as you sing or recite rhymes

Signing can also enrich language acquired through songs and rhymes. Singing and rhyming are very important tools for language learning. The rhythms and rhymes in songs and traditional nursery rhymes help babies learn and remember words and sounds. Many of the early childhood songs or nursery rhyme classics such as "Itsy Bitsy Spider," "Old MacDonald," "Hey Diddle Diddle," or "Little Miss Muffet" help babies acquire language skills. When you sing songs, don't worry that you don't have a great voice. Your baby doesn't care. She is mesmerized by the sounds and rhythm of the song. If songs are too uncomfortable for you, break out the Mother Goose nursery rhymes you remember from childhood or can find in books.

When you add signs to the songs you are singing or the rhymes you are repeating, you give your baby a multisensory learning experience. This deepens the learning experience and helps further develop your baby's mind. Sign the signs you know and don't worry about signing every word. You and your baby will have a great time while learning and increasing your bond.

Release your inhibitions and **SING** with your baby. Sing your favorite songs or opt for the baby classics such as "Itsy Bitsy Spider" and "Old MacDonald." Both of these are really good songs to sing and sign. When you sing "Itsy Bitsy Spider," sign **SPIDER, UP, WATER, DOWN, RAIN, SUN,** and **DRY**. When you sing "Old MacDonald," sign the animal signs. "Old MacDonald" is a wonderful way to introduce signs such as **DOG, CAT, DUCK, COW, HORSE,** and **PIG**.

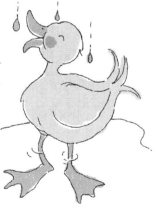

Sign sequences

Most parents want to get their baby into a routine. It is easier for both you and your baby when you have established patterns that are predictable and easy to follow. Children thrive when they know what's coming next. Signing can help you establish these patterns; you can explain to your baby what is going to happen next so things are not a surprise for her.

Sign sequences of events so she will learn routines and understand transitions. Here are three examples:

☆ Bedtime Routine: "First we will **EAT,** then you will take your **BATH,** then put on your **PAJAMAS,** then we will **READ** you a **BOOK**."

☆ Transitioning Activities: "We need to go **INSIDE** now because it is time to **EAT** dinner."

☆ Required Transition: "As soon as I **CHANGE** your **DIAPER** you can **PLAY MORE**."

As your baby grows and matures, signing a sequence of events will help you and your baby avoid meltdowns and misunderstandings because you will explain what is going to happen next. She will understand the sequence and be ready to make the changes that are coming. She will also be more patient when she needs to sit still for something like a diaper change because she knows that following the change, she will be able to play again.

AHA!

Karen's daughter heard music when Karen didn't even notice it. She would be in the store and find her daughter bouncing to the music that her mother had tuned out. Karen would then say, "Oh, you hear the **MUSIC**. I didn't even notice it. Let's **LISTEN** to the **MUSIC**." If you find your baby likes to move to music, suggest that you both **DANCE** to the music. Showing your baby how to move to the rhythms of music can help her with basic skills used later when learning math, such as relational and spatial skills and division and fractions (even Pythagoras identified music with numbers, noting its scales, tempos, and other regularities).

Use your baby's desire for MORE

As your baby learns about the world around her, she will want to repeat experiences and will likely use the sign **MORE** to help her get what she wants. For your baby, **MORE** can also mean "again," as in "Read that book again (**MORE**)." She might also use **MORE** to indicate that she wants you to keep tickling her or bouncing her. When you are playing, stop and ask her, "Do you want **MORE** bounces?" Wait for her to respond with a sign or with a body movement or smile. Then continue. As she gets older, wait longer so that she can independently ask you for what she wants.

Mealtime is also a good time to use the sign **MORE**. You can say, "Oh, that **CEREAL** is so yummy. Do you want some **MORE**? Let's have some **MORE CEREAL**." Then give your baby more cereal (see illustration.) But wait a bit to give her the next bite. By having to wait, your baby might have the incentive she needs to make her first sign. Often, parents find that the first sign their baby makes is **MORE** and that they make it when they want more food. Don't make your baby mad, but hesitate a bit and see whether she will ask you for more. Your baby will often make a sign when she needs something.

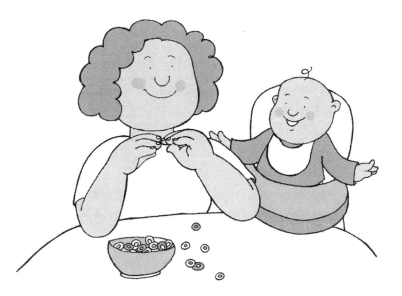

Make sure that you sign **MORE** in several contexts. If you only sign **MORE** when you feed your baby or when you read a book, your baby begins to associate the sign with that context only. Use **MORE** when you are asking "Do you want to stay in the bath longer?" (**MORE BATH**). **MORE** is a very versatile sign and can help your baby express her desires to you. Julie says, "I remember Zach's first sign. He was about thirteen months. We had only started doing signing about two months prior. My mother-in-law was bouncing him on her leg, and he signed **MORE MORE** very enthusiastically. We were all thrilled!"

One way to teach the concept of **MORE** is to gather something that you have a lot of, such as balls, spoons, blocks, or stuffed animals and play with them with your baby. Then hide them all from your baby's sight and then bring out one. Ask your baby whether she wants **MORE BLOCKS**. Bring out another one and exaggerate your excitement. Keep going, asking whether she wants **MORE** each time and making each block's appearance an exciting event. Your baby will be entertained and will learn the concept of **MORE** in a different way. Then say, "Wow, we have **A LOT** of **BLOCKS** to play with!"

Common Questions and Concerns about Signing

Invariably, in your signing experience you will have a few moments when you have questions or concerns. Here are the most common situations and how to best approach them.

Could that be a sign?

Your baby's first sign may not be perfect. Parents often wonder whether that hand squeeze was actually a sign or not. In one class I taught, a mother claimed that her nine-month-old, Ila, had never made a sign. As she was discussing this and saying that she signed **MILK** constantly, but Ila did not respond, the class broke into laughter because Ila signed **MILK** every time her mother mentioned the word. She had just turned her hand horizontal instead of vertical, so her mother thought she was waving instead of signing. But it was obvious that Ila was signing **MILK** because she made the sign only when her mother said "milk."

It may not actually matter whether Ila's hand movement was intended to be a sign, because babies learn through association. Research indicates that when a mother responds to random babbles, her baby's vocalizations become more advanced. What this means is that if your baby says "da, da," when Dad is in the room, you will find yourself saying "Do you see *Dad*?" Your baby might not have meant to say "Dada," as in Dad, but the association is starting to be made in your baby's head: the sound "dada" and that big, hairy guy that bounces me on his knee are connected. The same thing is true for signing. If you assign meaning to movements your baby makes, your baby will begin to make the association that these movements have meaning.

In fairness to Ila's mom, she might have missed Ila's first signs, because Ila was making an *approximation*. Look for motions that can be a sign. For example, your baby might wave her hand or reach out for the bottle when she wants **MILK**. She might put her hand in her mouth or point with one finger to her lips when she wants to **EAT**. Or she might sign **MORE** by clapping her hands or pointing one finger on the palm of her other hand or tapping her fists together. All of these approximations are common. Ask your baby, "Did I just see you sign **MORE**? Do you want some **MORE** banana?" Keep signing the signs correctly and your baby's signing ability will grow with her.

She's signing but I don't understand

If you do not understand what your baby is trying to sign, don't ignore her efforts. Instead, you can direct the conversation and try and figure out what she wants. For example, when you are eating and she is signing something you don't understand, speak to her and ask "Do you want some **BANANA**?" while you are signing the correct sign for banana. Then watch her reaction. She may show you that you got her request by her smile or excitement or she may even sign back the right sign.

The first sign—the same sign for everything

You may find that once your baby makes her first sign back, she will concentrate on that sign for several weeks. This is okay and is nothing to worry about. Your baby has just conquered a major milestone. The first sign is as precious as the first sounds your baby makes. It is the key to the entire signing game. You might even see her babbling it to herself with her fingers like babies babble spoken words to themselves.

Your baby might even use the same sign for several words. Don't worry. She is just working out the language process and is not confused. She has learned that when she squeezes her hand (**MILK**), you give her a bottle or nurse her. Her need is met. She may try to use the same **MILK** sign to get a cracker. She probably knows the difference between the two words, but she might not have the motor skills to make a sign for **CRACKER.** This is not surprising when you think about how babies learn spoken language. They often have a few sounds that they use for the words they want to say and use these sounds to try to communicate the things they want to say.

For example, your baby might use the sound "ba" for ball, baby, and bottle or "da" for daddy, dog, and doll. You'll understand her in context. If your baby is using the same sign for several things, keep signing the correct signs to your baby, and she will work out the language game and begin to understand that each specific object has its own sign. If she is receptive, help her form the correct sign. She will soon begin to differentiate the signs.

Respect any efforts your baby makes to interact, no matter how incorrect the sign or word may be. If, for example, your baby signs **MILK** horizontally instead of vertically, don't ignore her until she gets it right and don't say, "You're not signing that correctly." Acknowledge

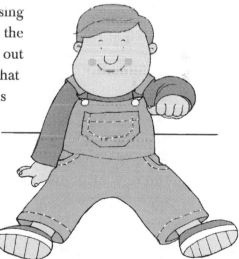

Some babies sign **MILK** with their hand turned sideways.

her sign and continue to make the sign correctly yourself without correcting her directly. "You would like some **MILK**? Let me get it for you." The same holds true for your baby's first words. Support any attempts your baby makes to vocalize and say words.

You don't know the sign or there is no sign

You may find that your baby requests signs from you that you do not know. Don't stress out. Just learn signs as you go along. For example, if your baby shows interest in a book that has pictures of animals, and you don't know all the signs, don't get flustered. Just take your baby's interest as a request for you to learn the signs. Check Part II for the signs and be prepared the next time you read that book.

Another way to react when you don't know a specific sign is to think of an alternative sign, such as a category sign or a question. Is the object a **VEGETABLE, FRUIT, ANIMAL,** or **TOY**? Adults often get hung up on knowing the specific sign for something. Your baby won't be frustrated if you sign **VEGETABLE** for asparagus or avocado or **FRUIT** for peach and plum. By signing the category sign for the new word your baby is learning, you are also helping her associate this thing with other things she knows that are similar. In the long run, this helps her understand the new word and increases her knowledge base.

If you are reading a book and don't know the sign for giraffe, say, "Look at how tall that **ANIMAL** is. It is called a giraffe." Then learn the sign for **GIRAFFE**. The next time you are reading, add the sign: "That tall **ANIMAL** is called a **GIRAFFE**. Where is the **GIRAFFE**? Can you point to it for me?" Or ask a question or make a comment such as **WHERE, WHAT, HELP, MORE, PLAY,** and **ALL DONE**. You could ask your baby, "**WHERE** is the giraffe? Show me" and have your baby point to the giraffe. If your baby does not know what a giraffe is, you can still ask the question and then help her point to the giraffe.

Some words are finger spelled in ASL, meaning their names are spelled out using the manual ASL alphabet. Don't be intimidated by finger spelling. If you come across words that need to be finger spelled, try it. The hearing babies of deaf parents do fine with finger spelled words, and many hearing parents who sign with their babies find that it works with them as well. However, if finger spelling scares you, there are ways to get your point across without finger spelling. You can use a general sign for the grouping of the sign you need. You can use the general sign **ANIMAL** if you don't want to finger spell armadillo or aardvark. If your baby likes a food that is finger spelled, sign **FOOD**.

Another solution is to create something called a *home sign*. A home sign is a sign that a family uses inside their own home that other people might not know. Home signs are similar to the baby talk parents sometimes use with their children. Some parents call the bottle a baba or a favorite blanket a lovey. These words may not make sense outside the family, but the baby and the parents understand. Creating a home sign works much the same way. If there is not a sign for something that your child needs a sign for, create a home sign. My son, for example, loved guacamole. I looked in every dictionary that I had and asked my deaf friends, and everyone told me that it was a finger spelled word. Guacamole is a long word to finger spell for a twelve-month-old. Instead of finger spelling it, we created a home sign.

AHA!

If your baby has favorite books that she loves to read, but that have signs you have a hard time remembering, make a cheat sheet for yourself and place it in the book or near the place you read books. If you are reading **The Very Hungry Caterpillar** and you cannot remember the signs for all the more obscure foods such as **PICKLE** (and you want to sign them), a cheat sheet can help you remember.

Note: ASL purists may be very adverse to parents' creating a home sign or not worrying about finger spelling. It's important to remember, however, that if parents get frustrated by finger spelling and stop signing altogether, their children are losing out on a good introduction to ASL, and a chance to communicate with their parents. It is better that parents do what is comfortable for them rather than stop signing because they are afraid.

Someday, these parents may feel comfortable enough to finger spell. Megan was one such mom. She started signing with her baby when Ella was eight months old. At first, she thought she would learn only five to ten signs, but as she and Ella learned to sign, she learned more and more. She and Ella used a few home signs for foods that Ella loved, such as yogurt. Then, to Megan's surprise, she met a new neighbor, Sara, who was deaf. Megan and Sara became great friends. Megan went on to learn ASL and interpret for her neighbor at times. As Megan explains, "I was really afraid of finger spelling when I started signing with my daughter. I just could not face it. But when I met Sara, I was ready. Signing with my daughter helped me feel comfortable enough to learn more ASL. I now have a great friend."

Your baby creates her own signs

You might find that your baby creates her own signs when she does not know a sign for something. This is a great insight into how children acquire language, and it is a common step in the process of gaining language. Julie's fourteen-month-old son, Jake, makes his own signs. "He'll look me in the eye and start signing away, looking like a third-base baseball coach doing all kinds of meaningful gestures, but I have no idea what he's saying, because I don't know those signs! It's clear he's trying to tell me something, and that he's used to me understanding his gestures, and doesn't quite get why I don't understand him when he does this. One of the most recent times he did this, he even repeated them more slowly trying to get me to understand him. I have managed to figure out that when he points up in the air he's saying 'outside' so I'm learning."

Your baby may be approximating a sign that is hard for her to make. Sheia's twelve-month-old son, Kyler, signed **CRACKER** by knocking his fist on his head because he could not figure out how to knock his fist on his elbow. Once you figure out what your baby is signing, make sure that you validate her efforts to communicate with you. If there is an actual sign for the thing your baby is signing, show her the real sign and help her form it in her hand. If there's not a sign for that thing, you can accept your baby's made-up sign as a home sign and use it. This shows her that she is an integral player in the language process.

Your baby doesn't sign back

A few parents have come to me claiming that their baby just doesn't like to sign. As we discussed the situation, I invariably find out that these parents are inconsistent in signing and can go for weeks without signing with their babies. No wonder their babies don't sign back. Make sure that even if you sign only a few signs, you sign consistently, so that your baby learns that she can trust that you are willing to communicate with her.

Some parents don't give their baby time to sign back. Mom and dad might be good at guessing what baby needs, but, even though they sign to the baby, they don't wait to get the response back. If you say, "Do you want some **MORE CEREAL**?" and then just give more cereal to your baby without waiting for her to respond back, what reason does she have to respond? Be patient. Sometimes the best learning comes when your baby wants something, and realizes that if she wants it, she can ask for it. You don't need to get her frustrated, but the time between wanting something and getting it can be a golden moment for you to ask for a sign and wait for it. Give her a chance to respond to you.

If you have been consistent in signing and your baby has still not signed back, don't give up. Sometimes your baby will start signing only to stop or sign erratically. Don't worry. As babies develop, they are constantly learning, and sometimes signing takes a backseat to the other things they have on their minds, such as crawling or walking. Tammy shared the following: "I had been signing to my daughter since she was five months with no response. She is now almost eleven months and just this past week she mastered walking. She started signing the same week!" Keep signing and speaking and your baby will continue to sign after she conquers the next milestone.

Even if your baby does not sign back, the added linguistic input from signing helps her learn language and will help her to speak. I have never heard of a baby who did not sign back if the parents signed with their baby consistently. Unless your baby has a physical or cognitive issue that would hinder her progress, she will sign. If she does have a physical or cognitive issue, see Chapter Eight for suggestions on how to adapt signing to her specific situation. Even some children with cerebral palsy respond to sign.

Signs for Eight to Twelve Months

You and your baby will be learning a lot of signs now and during the next eight to ten months. The following sections break down the signs that you may need to know at this age by the activities in which you will be using them. Once again, the signs shown here are also included in Part II, so that you can have an entire grouping of the signs that are appropriate for different activities. Copy and post the signs that you need in the appropriate locations. For example, post new meal signs on the fridge or near the high chair. Put new bath signs in the bathroom and activity signs where you play most.

Note: The signs listed here are not meant to be prescriptive. If you and your baby want to learn other signs, go right ahead. The best way to increase your communications is to sign things your baby is interested in.

Meal signs

This period is a great time to introduce your baby to a wide variety of foods. Babies are scientists by nature. But be prepared. This science experiment can have messy outcomes. Continue using the signs **MILK**, **MORE**, **EAT**, and **ALL DONE** that you were using previously. As you follow the suggestions of your pediatrician for what foods to introduce to your baby, you will gain a whole new topic to sign with your baby. When you are ready to feed your baby, say "Do you want to **EAT**? I have some **FOOD** for you. Let's sit down and **EAT**." If you sign **EAT** every time you feed your baby, you introduce the sign for both **EAT** and **FOOD**, because they are the same sign.

You should be introducing foods one at a time and waiting two to three days before introducing something new. This is a golden opportunity to introduce the sign for each food. Your baby's first food was probably cereal, but since then, you have probably started offering her a few tablespoons of vegetables or fruit in the same meal as a cereal feeding. Good foods to start with include sweet potatoes, squash, applesauce, bananas, carrots, peaches, and pears. Introduce your baby to the sign for each new food she tries.

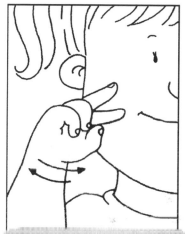

VEGETABLE: Twist index and middle finger at the side of the mouth

You might find that you don't know a sign for a specific vegetable or fruit. Just use the generic sign **VEGETABLE** or **FRUIT** until you learn the sign or learn to finger spell the word. If you begin feeding your baby chicken and beef, you can also use the general sign for **MEAT,** as babies don't necessarily need to differentiate chicken from beef. Even parents who do not sign with their children find that everything ends up as chicken. Monica says, "My son will eat anything we call chicken, but if I call the same thing beef, he will not eat it even if he likes it. So, we use the sign **MEAT** for all protein and that solves our problem."

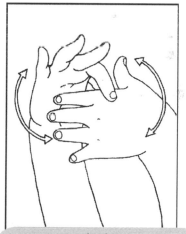

MEAT: Pinch skin between thumb and index finger and wiggle pinching hand

TWO CENTS

Your baby is also learning to use a spoon. This can make for some difficult signing moments. My son tried to use a spoon and sign at the same time. He forgot to put the spoon down first and ended up with applesauce on the side of his face. Don't worry. Just have fun with the signing at mealtime.

You will find that signing helps reduce the frustration babies feel as they begin to differentiate the foods they like and want. Carrie had been signing several different food signs with her son Nicholas. He had made a few signs back, but generally he signed **EAT** when he wanted food. One day, Carrie sat Nicolas down for lunch. She had fixed him a bowl of applesauce. Carrie knew he was hungry, but he would not eat the applesauce and started to get fussy. Carrie says, "I kept saying 'You love **APPLES**. Let's **EAT** some **APPLES**,' but he would not eat. Finally, he looked at me with a look that said, 'Mom you don't understand.' Then he signed **BANANA** and pointed to the bananas on the counter. If he had not been able to sign, I would never have understood why he would not eat or what he wanted. We probably would have had a big crying session." Carrie quickly got Nicholas the banana he requested and a crisis was averted.

For the most part, babies drink **MILK**, **WATER**, and **JUICE**. Milk is still coming from either a bottle or nursing. Use this sign as you have been using it previously. Introduce the signs for **WATER** and **JUICE** or **DRINK** when you introduce your baby to a sippy cup. This is a great way to transition to the cup. It is easier for babies to sign **DRINK**, so consider using this sign and the generic word "drink" for anything that is not water or milk. If you want to sign **JUICE**, don't worry. Your baby will

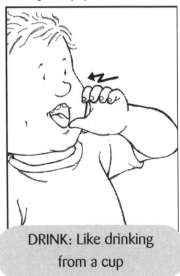

DRINK: Like drinking from a cup

approximate the sign while she cannot use just her pinkie. Her sign will probably end up looking a lot like **DRINK**.

Diaper/Dressing signs

Your baby is getting more mobile and does not want to stop. This makes diapering a dicey situation. Just when you have your baby lying down with the diaper open, and you are reaching for the wipes to clean off her poopy bottom, she decides it is time to get going. Not a situation that you want to be in. A few simple signs can help your baby understand that diapering is a time to sit still and that it won't last forever. This understanding won't come overnight, but you can start now and give you and your baby a way to communicate about what is happening.

You've probably already learned the sign **CHANGE** and you are signing to your baby when you are going to change her diaper. Continue to let her know what is going to happen. Babies, like everyone else, like to know what is going to happen to them. Do this by saying, "We're going to **CHANGE** your diaper. Let's go **CHANGE** that diaper. I am going to lay you **DOWN**." If your baby tries to get up, you can say, "You need to **WAIT**. Stay **DOWN**. I need to **CHANGE** your diaper." Then when you are finished, say, "We are **ALL DONE**. **THANK YOU** for waiting for me to **FINISH**. Let's get **UP** and get going!" The same signs work for babies who can't wait to be dressed and get back to playing. Let her know that you are going to **GET DRESSED** and then let her know when you are **ALL DONE** and that she can play now.

AHA!

Make sure you tell your baby what you *want* her to do and not what you don't want her to do. Children have a hard time understanding the concept of doing the opposite. Instead of saying "Don't get up," say "Stay down."

Activity signs

Continue using the signs suggested in Chapter Three. You will find that you have more activity time to interact with your baby now, and more chances to use these signs. If you have noticed that your baby has a preference for a few toys, learn the signs for these toys. Some of the best signs to learn are **DOLL**, **CAR**, **TRAIN**, **TELEPHONE**, **AIRPLANE**, and **BALL**. You can play with the toys and say and sign them to your baby. For example, if you have a toy telephone, say "Look at Mommy. She is talking on the **TELEPHONE**. Hello. Oh, you want to speak to Erika. The **TELEPHONE** is for you." By interacting in creative role play with your baby, you help increase her language skills.

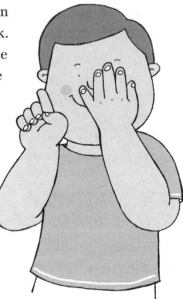

Your baby is also ready to engage in games like Peekaboo and Hide-and-Seek. Be careful because your baby may have separation anxiety, so don't hide where she cannot see you. Put a blanket over your head and let her pull it off or hide behind a door, where she can see most of your body, including your hands. Ask her, "**WHERE** is **DADDY**?" Or cover your eyes so you can't see her. Ask yourself, "**WHERE** is **BABY**?" You'll be surprised at how long your baby can play this game—probably for much longer than you will have interest in playing it.

Your baby is also beginning to experiment with cause and effect. She now notices what happens when she throws, drops, or shakes something. She will also seek the source of sounds. You can play a kind of sound hide-and-seek with her. Ask her, "What do you **HEAR**? What is that? **WHERE** is the sound coming from? Let's **LISTEN** again to see where the noise is coming from." Additionally, she might decide to make the noise herself. Your baby may smile with glee when she makes noise banging a spoon on her high chair or clapping two pan lids together. You can respond by saying, "This is very **LOUD**. You have learned to make a lot of **NOISE**."

Safety signs

There are several signs that you can show your baby to help her stay safe and stay away from things that are off limits. One of the first signs you can show your baby is **NO TOUCH**. She will often be in situations where there are things that are off limits. You can only show this sign in context. When you see your baby going for something she should not touch, because it is dangerous or she could break it, remove her hand and get her attention and clearly explain, "**DO NOT TOUCH** that." As your baby gets older, she might test the limits of what is a **NO TOUCH**. Make sure that you always react the same way—clear and direct—this is a **NO TOUCH** situation.

When your baby is interacting with other children or animals, **SOFT TOUCH** is an excellent sign to show her. Your baby may not know that she could hurt an animal or another baby. When you see her moving toward the cat, say "Use a **SOFT TOUCH**" and

AHA!

Follow your baby's lead in play. When she is ready to stop, stop. If she wants more, play more. Remember to take turns. She learns to engage in play if you wait and give her time to respond during games. If she prefers a certain game or book, that is great. You may tire of the repetition, but the important thing is that you are interacting.

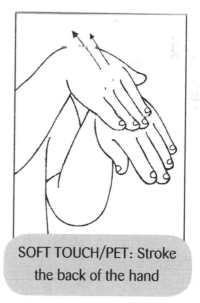

SOFT TOUCH/PET: Stroke the back of the hand

take her hand and show her how to softly touch the cat. But just because you say and sign **SOFT TOUCH** doesn't mean that she understands how she should pet the cat. Demonstrate to her how to pet the cat and say, "See how Mommy uses a **SOFT TOUCH** with the cat? The cat likes it when I touch her softly." You can underscore this lesson during playtime by taking your baby's bear and saying, "Oh, **TEDDY** likes it when I use a **SOFT TOUCH**. Can you touch **TEDDY** with a **SOFT TOUCH**?" If you give your baby massages, use this time to underscore the concept of **SOFT TOUCH**. When you massage her, say "I am using a **SOFT TOUCH**."

WAIT, **STOP**, and **HELP** will give her additional ways to understand what she can and can't do. If you need her to wait for a while, say "Please **WAIT**. We need to change your diaper." Don't expect that she will understand this right now, but she will grow into understanding the concept of waiting. Use the sign **STOP** instead of saying no, which babies often ignore. For example, if she is reaching for something that is off limits, say and sign **STOP** to help her know that it is off limits.

When you can see that your baby needs help doing something, ask her "Do you need some **HELP**? I will come **HELP** you." With time she will request your help. The **HELP** sign is difficult for babies to make until they are well over a year old. So when you see that she needs help, offer your help to your baby. When she does want to ask for help, she might grunt or look up to you to ask for help. She might also approximate the sign. Often, babies will sign **HELP** by tapping two hands on their chest. Without teaching them to do this, I have seen dozens of babies make this exact approximation. Take advantage if your baby does tap on her chest and ask, "May I **HELP** you?"

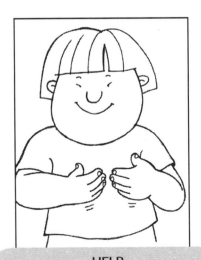

HELP
Since **HELP** is difficult to sign, many babies will tap their chest to indicate, "**HELP**."

A final sign that is very important to a baby's safety is **HURT**. Your baby may need to tell you that she has been hurt. She might have fallen in her attempts to walk or she might have a new tooth that is emerging. With **HURT,** your baby can tell you where it hurts and help you diagnose the source of her tears. **HURT** is a very handy sign because you sign it wherever something hurts. If you have a **HEADACHE,** you sign **HURT** at your head. If you have an **EARACHE**, you sign **HURT** at your ear. If you have fallen and hurt your leg you sign **HURT** at the point where the scrape is. As your baby walks and gets more mobile and independent, this sign becomes more useful. Also, it helps when you have to go to the doctor for shots or other procedures.

Bath signs

Now that your baby is sitting up on her own in the bath, this becomes a wonderful place for her to play and explore. Let her splash in the tub and say, "Yes, you can make the **WATER** move. Splash, splash goes the **WATER**." If she has toys in the bath, show her the signs for them, such as **BOAT, DUCK**, and **BALL**. You can say, "Let's **PLAY** with your **BOAT**." However, don't be surprised if it is awhile before she plays with the toys in the bath. Just the experience of being in the bath is a lot for your baby to take in.

Show your baby the signs for **WASH**, **WASH HAIR**, and **CLEAN**. Your baby may really enjoy the process of getting clean and you can enhance this by signing and singing while she is in the bath. The old song "The Mulberry Bush" can be changed to "Wash our Baby."

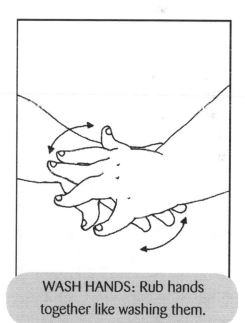

WASH HANDS: Rub hands together like washing them.

TWO CENTS

One of the best baby music CDs for bath time is Do-Rey-Me-and You's *Tub Tunes*. If you want to get bath time a-rockin', put this in before, during and after your baby's bath. You'll both be dancing to "Yellow Submarine," "Rub-a-Dub-Dub," and "Splish Splash"!

This is the way we **WASH** our baby **WASH** our **BABY, WASH** our baby This is the way we **WASH** our baby So early Monday morning.

This is the way we **WASH** our toes **WASH** our toes, **WASH** our toes This is the way we **WASH** our toes So early Tuesday morning.

You get the picture. Add verses for other body parts on other days of the week. You can even extend this to add in verses about getting dry, brushing teeth, brushing hair, and getting dressed. Be creative!

If your baby has a hard time having her hair washed, showing her the sign for **WASH HAIR** can help her understand that you are about to wash her hair. If her dislike for washing her hair continues, when she gets a bit older you can have her wash her doll's hair or watch you wash your hair. Or you can read a book about washing hair. If she sees the activity happening with other people, it might help her get over her fear. Make sure that when you are finished, you sign **ALL DONE** so that she knows the torture is over.

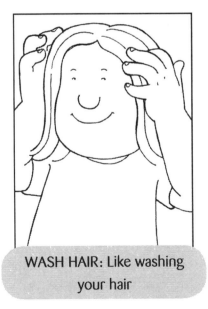

WASH HAIR: Like washing your hair

Bedtime signs

Your baby eventually needs to learn to sleep independently—to be able to fall asleep unassisted and put herself back to sleep if she wakes up. But this is often not an easy task, as evidenced by the shelves and shelves of books on this topic that are available at the bookstore. Whatever method you use to get your baby to sleep independently is your choice. There are some signs that can help you in this quest.

Sleep experts agree that having a nighttime ritual is one of the very best ways to prepare your baby for bed. You might read a **BOOK** or **SING** or take a **BATH**. Doing these activities in the same order each night helps your baby prepare herself for the separation from you. You can also use the signs **ALL DONE** and **LIGHTS OFF** to help her understand that this is the end of your ritual and it's time for her to transition to **SLEEP**.

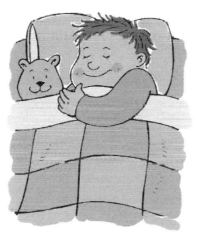

In our house, we always read *The Going to Bed Book* right before going to bed. The book progresses through an evening ritual for getting ready for bed. It even shows the **LIGHT** being turned **OFF.** This helped my son understand that everywhere the same things take place at bedtime. We memorized the book so when we would put him to bed, we would quote the lines from the book that corresponded to the activity we were doing. That way, he could associate what he saw in the book with what he was experiencing.

A Final Note on Staying Motivated

Many parents will stop signing with their babies or sign inconsistently if they are concentrating on the wrong thing. You are not "teaching" your baby something to show off at the family Thanksgiving meal. You are creating a relationship of communication with your baby. If you feel overwhelmed by signing, stop and take stock. What is your motivation? Are you trying to "teach" your baby instead of just using signs with your daily activities and conversations? Are you trying to do too much?

If you or your baby is stressed out by your attempts to sign, take a breather. Just keep signing five to eight signs and give yourself a rest. Then start adding signs back in when you feel comfortable again. Remember your goal—you want to communicate with your baby and help her communicate with you. You will be spending a lot of time together and you don't have to do everything in one day. If she is working on large motor skills such as crawling and walking and shows less interest in signing, just keep signing and she will begin to sign again when she has mastered her latest skill. You will both appreciate the ability to sign in the next several months, when her desire to express her independence and have her needs met grows exponentially.

Summary

In this chapter, we discussed:

    ☆ How your baby is developing from eight to twelve months

    ☆ What to expect from your baby's first signing attempts

    ☆ Strategies to increase your child's ability to sign

    ☆ Common questions and problems parents encounter

    ☆ Signs and activities to use in this period

Bottom Line

Your baby will probably sign back during this time or soon after her first birthday. Look for the first sign, because it may be hard to recognize. Don't worry if a few issues come up—signing is something you will incorporate into your daily life and is something you will be doing for the next year or so.

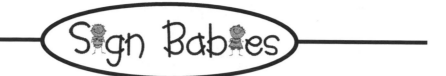

Chapter Five

Thirteen to Eighteen Months—I'm Ready for More, More, More

For most babies, the period from thirteen to eighteen months is a time of extensive movement and memory development. Your baby is now walking about freely, and is discovering the world around him. He has a lot to learn, and sometimes it seems like he wants to learn it all in one day.

During this time, his ability to remember things and recall information also increases greatly. He now knows that you will return when you leave him for a while. He understands that when his **BEAR** is not in his sight, it is somewhere else (*object permanence*) and that he can go look for it. His need to express his wants and desires is also growing during this time, outpacing his verbal abilities to express himself. Signing will help him communicate and keep his frustration to a minimum.

In this chapter, we'll take a look at the following:
★ How your baby is developing from thirteen to eighteen months
★ How reading helps his development

✰ How your baby's signing abilities will explode

✰ How your baby's independence can be influenced by signing

✰ Specific activities to use during this period

JUST BEGINNING NOW? If you are just starting to sign with your baby, read the previous chapters before you begin signing consistently. You will learn the signs that are best to start with and strategies for signing with your baby in various situations, such as reading books and eating dinner. You can expect your baby to sign as quickly as a week or two after you begin signing. The signs you start with may be different than if you signed with your baby earlier. Start with signs that will motivate your child, such as **FOOD** or **TOYS**, and other signs related to activities he enjoys.

Your Baby's Development

Your baby is now working on the big things such as walking, jumping, and talking. You might be surprised by how much your baby will change during this period.

Motor development

Walking is one of the most exciting events in early life for babies and their parents. A baby's first steps are just the beginning of a complex motor skill that continues to develop throughout the second year of life. By eighteen months, you will notice that his steps are smoother, landing first with the heel and moving to the toe. He will become more coordinated and will easily navigate around obstacles instead of tripping over them. Much of the improvement in motor development occurs because his brain now has more myelin—a dense, fatty substance that helps neurons send and receive messages faster and more clearly. Walking practice also helps his motor development by strengthening his muscles and improving his sense of balance. Provide lots of opportunities for him to practice his walking skills.

The same development of myelin also helps your baby's hand coordination, which means that he can sign more signs in this period than he could before. He now has the manual dexterity to sign a wider range of more complex signs involving two hands and slight movements. Where your baby's signs were once unclear and difficult to understand, they will become more distinct and specific, as well as more numerous.

Language development

Your baby's language abilities are growing quickly. You can now give him simple directions such as "Give me your **BOOK**," and he can comply. *Whether* he will comply is a different matter. Some babies choose not to comply as a display of the independence they are now feeling. Babies are beginning to understand their autonomy from their parents at this age and this feeling of independence is often expressed by refusing to comply with a parental request.

You will find that your baby knows many signs and words. The average child who does not sign will be able to understand ten to fifteen frequently used words. Babies who sign with their parents can often sign at least this many signs, and often as many as one hundred signs. This means that your baby has the ability to understand ten times more words because you sign with him than if you did not sign with him. He can now easily point to a picture in a book when you ask him "**WHERE** is the . . . ?" and make the correct sign. He may even know how to say the word or make a sound associated with the word. Your baby will probably begin to enjoy language games that ask him to identify things. You can say and sign, "**WHERE** is your ear?" and "**WHERE** is Mommy?"

His vocabulary will grow quickly during this time, but his pronunciation can't keep pace. Fortunately he can sign and will quickly learn a lot of new signs during this time. If your baby does try to speak, resist the temptation to correct his pronunciation. Most babies mispronounce their words, and often babies will continue to sign words that they have learned to say because the pronunciation is so difficult. Just continue to speak and sign with your baby and use the correct pronunciation. This works better

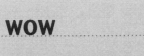

WOW

Ashell says, "Our cat was sitting in his stroller and Davis was standing in front of him and was holding up his hand and putting his forefinger and thumb together. I didn't recognize it as a sign at first. Then he did it again while he was chasing a cat. I finally realized that he was signing **CAT**. He made the association all by himself."

than correcting his pronunciation ever would. Your baby will eventually transition from signing to a signing/speech combination and finally to speech alone.

One other thing to remember is that your baby may try to communicate whole thoughts through single words or signs. **BALL**, for example, may mean "Look at the ball," "I want the ball," or "Where is the ball?" You can clarify this by asking your baby questions and looking at his other signals. For example, does he sign **SLEEP**, but shake his head no? He might be saying that he does not want to go to sleep. Your conversations will grow in complexity and interest for both you and your baby.

Cognitive development

The area of your baby's brain called the hippocampus, also referred to as "the seat of memory," has matured enough that it is possible for him to recall actions and events that occurred a few hours or even a day earlier. This (called *deferred imitation*) means that your baby has the potential to learn from what he sees others do. For example, one day you might show your baby a new sign that he does not repeat immediately. But he might display it in some form later in the day or week when you least expect it.

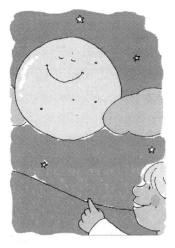

You may be surprised by what your baby can recall and when he chooses to recall things. It was during this time when my son signed **MOON** for the first time. We were outside and he started to moo like a cow. We live in the city and there are no cows nearby so I could not understand why he would moo. Then he looked at me as if to say, "Don't you get it, Mom?" and he signed **MOON**. He had never signed that sign. I had made the sign earlier in the week when we had been reading *Goodnight, Moon* but I had never made the sign to him outside when looking at the moon. He took the information from the book and applied it to real life and showed me the moon. We then started an evening ritual of going outside and saying goodnight to the moon.

Your baby loves to do the same activities over and over again—it is comforting to him. You are probably tired of reading the same baby book, playing the same game, or signing the same song. However, repetition is a very important learning tool for babies. When things repeat or have a consistent pattern, your baby learns to expect or anticipate the outcome. This is one reason why many baby books repeat the same structure or pattern. Once your baby learns the pattern, he can concentrate on learning the details such as the names of the animals. If you are playing a game over and over, he learns the rhythm of the game and learns to predict the outcome—a significant learning skill.

AHA!

You might want to evaluate whether or not you are using all the signs you have taught your baby. Have you stopped using some signs? Do you need to use a few more signs? By repeating the same signs you have been using, you are helping your baby learn more quickly. Add signs for things your baby is interested in because he will be more inclined to sign things he likes.

Embrace repetition. In some ways, it makes parenting easier. You don't have to know how to sing fifty songs and you don't have to come up with new activities all the time. Your baby will probably love the same few books no matter how extensive his choices are. Use repetition to your advantage when you want to show new signs. If you have been signing just a few signs when you read his favorite book, add in a few more. Because he is already familiar with the text, adding a new sign adds a dimension of learning for him based on what he already knows.

Social development

You may notice that your baby has a hard time controlling his feelings and emotions at this time—this is the onset of the Terrible Twos, which actually start in the middle of the second year of life, not after the second birthday. Toddlers face a high level of frustration at this age that usually stems from their inability to express their needs, desires, and intensifying emotions. Sometimes the frustration comes from not being able to do or have something they want. Signing will help your baby express his needs, wants, and feelings and should lessen the number of tantrums you experience.

Your baby is also just learning how to control his behavior, a skill called *inhibition*. Even if he knows that biting a friend is unacceptable, he may not be able to override the initial desire to bite. This is partially because inhibition is thought to be a function of the brain's frontal lobes, which are now undergoing a great deal of maturation. Additionally, if babies have no way to express themselves, their ability to control their behavior is limited. When a baby learns to sign and can express his feelings, he can begin to learn to control his behavior. Expressing how he feels and having you validate these feelings often can diffuse the situation and allow your baby to feel validated. You can then teach him constructive ways to deal with his emotions.

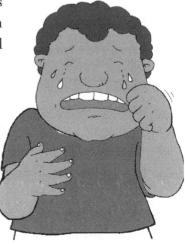

Give your child ways to express himself with language through sign and words. You can teach him signs such as **SAD**, **CRY**, and **HAPPY** to help him share his feelings. Then show him the rules of behavior. For example, you can say, "Michael, you can't **HURT** your sister, but you can tell her not to take (**NO TOUCH** or **STOP**) your toy." Remember that if your baby is tired, hungry, or upset, he may not be able to control himself. Look for signs of frustration before a situation gets out of hand and help your baby by making sure he gets enough rest, eats on schedule and has time to decompress. Over stimulation can be the cause of many tantrums.

Even though you give your baby ways to express himself through sign, a few tantrums will come. This is a natural process of learning that helps him learn to cope with and get through difficult situations. Sympathize with your baby when he has a meltdown. Let him know that the behavior is unacceptable, but that you still love him. This will give him the stability to learn to deal with his emotions and understand the rules. Make sure that the consequences of his actions are clear and appropriate for the situation.

WOW

Julia relates the following: "I received a phone call at work from my fifteen-month-old daughter's teacher. Her teacher said that Ruby was signing HURT at her mouth. When the teacher looked in her mouth, she had painful looking blisters in there. I can't begin to tell you how wonderful it is to have a baby who is able to communicate what is the matter at such a young age. I picked her up and was able to get her into the pediatrician that day."

The Importance of Reading

You are entering the golden age of book reading. Even though it might be hard for your baby to sit and listen, reading is really important. Literacy is one of the greatest gifts you can give your child. A lifelong love of books will open more doors for him than you can imagine. Don't worry if reading sessions only last a few minutes because your baby is so mobile. Experts suggest fifteen to twenty minutes of reading every day has long-term benefits for your baby's learning abilities. You can always change your reading time to when he is less mobile and more ready to sit and listen a bit.

Here are a few suggestions for engaging your baby in reading and adding new dimensions to your reading experiences:

✰ Start each reading time by inviting your baby to read. Over time, this sets up your baby's expectations for what the experience will be like.

✰ Designate a cozy spot for reading. We read in the big bed or in an oversized chair so all kids can see the book and enjoy some intimate time together.

✰ Choose books that you feel comfortable signing, but don't shy away from books you can't sign. You can ask questions such as "**WHERE** is the armadillo?" instead of knowing the sign for armadillo.

✰ Sign anything you know from the story and ask your baby to sign what he knows. If there is an animal you know the sign for, sign it. Signing makes reading an interactive experience. Your baby can comment on what he sees and participate in the reading.

✰ If the text is too hard for your baby, simplify and use the pictures to tell your own story.

✰ Choose books that interest your baby. If your baby loves airplanes, read books about airplanes. Remember, these books don't have to be interesting to you because you already know how to read.

✰ Choose books that correspond to rhymes or songs you use with your baby at other times. If your baby is familiar with the sound of the book, you can reinforce the signs you are using with him in the song or rhymes.

✰ Ask your baby questions about what is happening in the book. "Can you show me **WHERE** the turtle is?" or "What sound does the **CAT** make?" Your baby may not be able to answer you back clearly, but respond to what he does say and sign. His verbal and nonverbal responses are important stepping stones to greater literacy.

✰ Choose books whose pictures allow you to tell your own story. Books such as *Good Night Gorilla* and *Ten Minutes to Bedtime* have very few words. You can discuss the books with your baby and focus on things such as finding **WHERE** the mouse is on each page. You can sign the animals and make their sounds. Don't get stuck on armadillo. Just sign **ANIMAL**.

☆ Read books that have to do with activities you and your baby do often. For example, *The Going to Bed Book* is a great book for showing children the routine of getting ready for bed. Read this book right before bedtime and then act out the book by doing the activities the book talks about.

Not enough can be said about the power of reading fifteen to twenty minutes a day with your baby. Children gain lifelong learning skills through reading, such as:

☆ understanding the process of reading

☆ understanding reading left to right, turning pages

☆ understanding that stories have a beginning, middle and end

☆ becoming aware of letters

☆ understanding that letters and words have meaning

Research has shown that the effects of reading go well beyond just being able to read. A few of them include:

☆ increased listening skills

☆ increased attention span and memory

☆ increased vocabulary and understanding of words

☆ stimulation of the imagination and other senses

A complete list of the books suggested throughout this book as well as many others that can be signed is located in Appendix C. But it's okay if you read the same three to four books over and over again. Babies love repetition.

The Signing Explosion

Your baby now has the manual dexterity and cognitive abilities he needs to express what he needs with signs. He may also be speaking a few words, but it could be several months before he can communicate equally as well in speech as he can with sign. This is the time when most babies begin to explode with signs: They increase the number of signs they make and the contexts they use them in. They may also begin to use two sign combinations such as **MORE MILK**.

You can help your baby learn signs with a few of these strategies:

☆ Add sounds to your signs and words. When you sign animal signs, make the sound that the animal makes. For example, when you sign **ELEPHANT**, make a trumpeting sound. Or when you sign **TIGER**, growl. Making the sound helps your baby focus on what you are doing and helps him associate the sounds he has learned in other situations with the correct sign and the word.

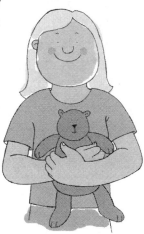

☆ Sign near or on the object you are signing about. If you have a stuffed animal such as a bear, make the sign for **BEAR** right on the bear (see illustration.) This helps your baby see the sign and the object it represents together. You can even add a bear growl.

☆ Sign the signs right on your baby. For example, if you are playing with a teddy bear while your baby is sitting on your lap, say, "Do you love your **BEAR**?" Sign **BEAR** right on your baby's chest.

☆ Set up a situation where your baby needs to make a choice. When you ask him whether he wants an **APPLE** or a **BANANA** to eat, you place him in a situation where he needs to communicate with you. He may choose to point or sign the fruit he wants. Either way, he is learning that communication gets him what he wants.

Make sure that you invite your baby to the conversation. You can even tap him on the hands and say "Let's talk about it." He may sign with you, but don't worry if he doesn't. He can talk to you through his body language—you should value this as much as a sign or a clear word. By inviting your baby to participate, you are teaching him that his opinions and responses matter.

IMPORTANT: One issue that arises during the signing explosion is that a lot of the signs your baby makes may look the same. This is because your baby's fine motor skills may not be advanced enough to make the fine distinctions between movements. You will generally be able to tell what the sign is in context. Jennifer discovered this with her son. "My eighteen-month-old son, Lucas signs more than forty signs and a lot of them look exactly the same. Just like when a mother knows what her own child is speaking when it sounds like gibberish to others, I know exactly what Lucas is signing based on context. For a long time, **BALL**, **MORE**, **HELP** and just clapping looked a lot alike. Also, for a while he made **MOM, GRANDMA, WATER** and **BIRD** all by pointing one finger to his mouth. Repeating what he says and signs with the correct word and sign is helping him to learn the correct signs. I love that he's communicating!"

ONLINE

Join the discussion about sign language online at the Sign Babies Web Site (www. signbabies.com). There are links to podcasts, videos, pictures and other resources for parents signing with babies.

Look for signing opportunities

As with anything you will introduce to your baby, timing is everything. If your baby is interested, happy, or calm, he will be more receptive to seeing and learning a sign than when he is tired or interested in something else. Look for the following clues for when your baby is ready to receive a sign:

☆ Is he staring at an object with interest? He might want to know more about it. This is a good time to introduce the sign for the object if you know it. For example, if he sees a dog walk by and stares at it, take the chance to say, "You see the **DOG**? Yes, that is a **DOG**."

☆ Did he move toward an object of interest? His movement is an outward expression of his interest. If he goes for a doll at a friend's house, say "Do you like that **DOLL**?" Then converse with him about the doll as he holds it.

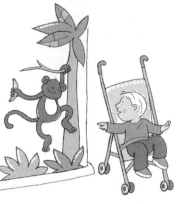

☆ Has his mood changed? Has he become intent or very excited about something? Introducing the sign can help him understand what he is excited about. For example, on a trip to the zoo, your baby sees his first **MONKEY**. He becomes very excited. Say to him, "That is a **MONKEY**. Can you see the **MONKEY** swinging on the branch?"

☆ Is he just about to get frustrated because he can't express himself or get what he needs? Sometimes the moment between the calm and the frustration is a perfect time to introduce a sign. If he sees you eating some cheese and you can tell he wants to try it, ask him, "Do you want to try the **CHEESE**?"

Your baby might reach out for a banana or a cracker or show you his excitement by jumping or wiggling when he sees a dog. Use these moments to introduce new signs or reinforce signs he already knows. Ask him, "Do you want **MORE BANANA**?" or "Did you see that **BIG DOG**?" In the first instance, you are reiterating two signs he already knows, but it may be the first time you have signed two signs together. In the second instance, you are adding a descriptor sign, **BIG**, to a sign he already knows, **DOG**. This expands his knowledge.

Going beyond just names

Close to his first birthday, your baby will realize that not only do things have names, but they also have functions. Instead of just chewing on the telephone, he will have a conversation with someone on the other end. He will take the spoon and stir the pot with it, not just bang with it.

When you see this behavior, it signals a great time to go beyond just labeling things and start telling your baby how things function or explaining what he is hearing, seeing, tasting, smelling or feeling (*parallel talk*). By doing so, you are increasing your baby's spoken and signing vocabulary and helping him learn other cognitive skills. When you are in the kitchen, give him a

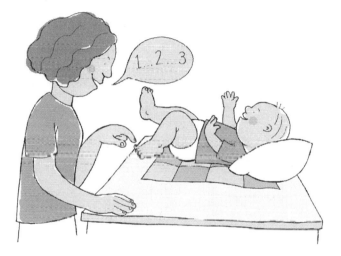

spoon and a pot and say, "Let's make something to **EAT**. Put the **SPOON** in the pot and stir the **SOUP**." Besides learning new words and signs, he is gaining understanding of the concept of making soup.

Interacting with your baby at this level can also set the stage for even more complex cognitive learning. For example, when you are changing your baby's diaper, you can tell him the names for the parts of the body. Then take it one step further. Count the number of fingers and toes he has (see illustration.) He probably won't start counting soon, but hearing the numbers helps him be prepared for counting sooner than you think.

I would always count my son's toes when we changed diapers or got dressed. When he was eighteen months old, we were in a mom and baby music class where there was a song and activity that included counting to

AHA!

Signing helps parents use key labeling words instead of abstract pronouns—a key to language learning success. When you sign, you ask your baby "**WHERE** are your **SHOES**?" not "Where are they?" This helps him know what you are asking him to find. Parents who don't sign may not make this subtle change in their language and may have less successful interactions with their babies.

five. The teacher did not expect the babies to count, but was doing the activity as a precursor to later skills. After the song, we had free time. My son began pulling shells out of the basket and laying them on the floor while counting out loud as he placed them on the floor—one, two, three, four, five. The teacher noticed this and came and watched. He did this several times. She commented that he was repeating the exercise from the song.

But then he did something unexpected. He removed only three shells and counted them one, two, three. Then he removed two shells and counted them one, two. Then he removed four shells and counted them correctly as well. He had understood more than just the repetition of the exercise. He had understood the concept that the objects had a value assigned to them in their grouping. The teacher was amazed because this is a cognitive skill that most children conquer well past their second birthday.

Conversing with your baby

Your goal is to have conversations with your baby—to use sign language to help bridge the time before he can speak so that you can start to communicate now. This also means that you should be talking to your baby often. For parents, talking to their baby is sometimes difficult because they don't know how to talk to someone who can't really talk back.

Here are three ways you can have a conversation even when he can't talk back.

Parallel talk is talking about what you see. You describe what your baby is doing. He can hear the words that go with the activities he is participating in: "You are **PLAYING** with the **DOLL**. Does your **BABY** want some **MILK**?"

Self talk is talking about what you are doing. Your baby watches you and what you are doing: "I am **WASHING** my hands. Now I am **COOKING** dinner." When you narrate what you are doing, you give him words and signs for the things he sees you do.

Stretch talk or *expansion* is adding to what your baby is saying or signing. If he signs **EAT,** you say, "You want to **EAT**? How about some **APPLES**? Let me put some **APPLES** on your plate." You have stretched his request for food and added a specific type of food, apples, and a place to put the food, a plate.

He will use the words he learns through parallel talk, self talk, and stretch talk later when he is ready to talk about similar things. His first sentences in sign and speech will be *telegraphic*, meaning that they will leave out words such as "a" and "the." **MORE DRINK** is a common example.

Combining signs and adding descriptors

Your baby's ability to communicate is becoming more and more sophisticated. If you have not already done so, now is a great time to start combining more than one sign in your conversations.

You will also find that your baby begins to sign multiple signs to express himself. He can sign **MORE BANANA** to let you know that he wants to eat more bananas. Most of his first two sign combinations will include **MORE** and another sign. Babies want more of everything and this is an easy way for him to express his need. **MORE** also may mean "again," as in **MORE BOOK,** which can translate to "Read that book to me again, please."

He also may sign combinations such as **PLAY BALL** when he wants to play with the ball or **BABY CRY** if he hears another baby cry. You will be surprised at what your little one can tell you and how early these two sign combinations will appear. My daughter Anna signs **DADDY BATH** when she wants her dad to give her a bath.

Talk with your baby and have conversations with him even when he cannot answer back. You are basically commenting on the things around you. Toward the end of this period is a good time to add descriptive signs to the list of signs your baby already knows. For example, when he sees a **DOG,** comment that it is a **BIG DOG** or a **LITTLE DOG**. You can also add colors to your conversations.

Say, "See the **YELLOW FLOWER**? It is called a rose." You are giving him the name for the color of the flower and the name of the flower itself. With time, he will be able to tell you descriptive things about his world, but this may not happen until after he is two years old. As he gets older, continue to add descriptors so that his receptive language skills strengthen. Just do not expect that he will understand them all for some time.

Dealing with Your Baby's Independence

Babies have a need to do things themselves. Some babies start earlier than others, but they all want the independence to do things on their own. As a parent, you know that your baby cannot feed himself or clean his own face or throw the ball well without your help. However, you don't want to squelch his independence by always doing for him what he has not mastered. If he is really set on doing something, a temper tantrum and power struggle can occur. Or, if he is passive about it, your baby will learn to let you do it for him and may come to expect you to do it all the time.

Even though it is messy, you want your baby to learn to do things on his own. Signing can help you balance his need for independence with his need to be helped. When he is learning to use a spoon, tell him you are going to **TAKE TURNS**. He can use the spoon to eat one bite (his **TURN**) and then you are going to feed him one bite (**MOMMY'S TURN**). When he is in the bath and you want him to stop playing in the water and wash his body, engage him by asking him for his help. Say "**HELP** Mommy, please. We are going to **WASH** you and I need your **HELP**." When you solicit his help, he feels that he is independent and capable.

If your baby will not do something that you want him to do, try doing it yourself at the same time. If he will not eat, take a bite of your food and say in an exaggerated tone, "Oh, I love to **EAT**. Yummy. Do you want some? **NO**? Okay. I am going to **EAT MORE.** Yum!" Or, if your baby doesn't want to get dressed, get dressed along with him. "Mom is going to put on her **CLOTHES**. See, I have my shirt on. Do you want to **TAKE** a **TURN**?" This also works when you need to get out the door and your baby will not let you put on his shoes, gloves, coat, or hat. Try to **TAKE TURNS** and see if he gives in.

AHA!

Ask your baby if you can **TAKE** a **TURN** with a toy. You are showing him the beginning skills he needs to **SHARE**. Take a toy that you know your baby likes to play with but is not playing with at the moment. If he gets interested, say, "Oh, would you like a **TURN** to play with the doll? Here you go?" Let him play with it for awhile and then ask, "Can **MOMMY** have a **TURN**? May I play with the doll?" If he does not give it to you, don't worry. Sharing and taking turns are high level cognitive functions that he might not be ready for until 3 years old. You are setting the stage for future skills.

IMPORTANT: Don't give your child an option if you really need him to do something. This applies in all situations. If you need him to do something or you must do something, make a statement: "We are going to the store." Don't say: "Do you want to go to the store?" If you ask a question, you are implying choice. If there is no choice, don't ask it as a question.

Encouraging signing instead of screaming

During this age, your baby's need to get specific things he wants increases. He now understands that there are specific things he wants and likes. For many parents, this begins the unhappy odyssey of trying to guess what it is that their baby wants. For parents who do not sign with their babies, this may mean a lot of screaming and head scratching—screaming on the baby's part and head scratching on the parent's part. When you show your baby the signs for the things he wants, you have a way to bypass the frustration.

As your baby's need to express himself increases in parallel with his growing independence and desire to learn about his world, there will be many instances where he needs to communicate something to you. You have taught your baby to sign to help him explain his needs, but he will not always remember that he has the skill, and he may start to cry. Whenever you sense that he wants something but can't get his point across, ask him to "Tell me with your hands (**SIGN**)." This might help him remember that he knows how to communicate with you in a more effective manner than screaming.

You can also use "Tell me with your hands (**SIGN**)" for times when he tries to use spoken words but they are not clear. Tricia read to her son Dallin every day before nap time. "When he was eighteen months old, he was starting to replace signs with words and was trying to tell me something that he wanted. I did not understand. He looked up at me disgusted and signed **BOOK**." He was ready for his book and his nap. Without the

WOW

Your baby can sign to tell you things you may not know. Sara says that her son Gabe was crying like he was in pain. She started to check him to see whether he had hurt himself. "I asked him where it HURT and he looked at me and signed HURT by his teeth. I understood right away that he was getting a new tooth and got the numbing gel to help him. If he had not been able to sign HURT, it might have been much harder for me to understand that he was teething."

sign, Dallin probably would have broken into tears. By helping your baby to realize that he has a way to clarify his point and ensure that he is getting it across, you can skip many of the tantrums caused when children feel they are powerless to get what they need.

Introducing good manners

Many child development books say that children cannot learn good manners until they are close to three years old. Parents who sign with their babies have an advantage and can start to help their babies understand and use good manners much earlier. Start to show your baby the signs that will help him have good manners and play well with other children by using these signs yourself when you speak with him. This is called *modeling*. Babies learn by example, so when you speak with your baby, say such things as, "**PLEASE** may I **PLAY** with your **DOLL**?" or "**THANK YOU** for helping me **CHANGE** your diaper."

It may sound strange to talk this way, but it does two things. It introduces your baby to the language of good manners, and it gives him a chance to feel the effects of good manners. When you treat your baby with respect and ask him if you can play with his doll and thank him for his cooperation when changing diapers, you respect his individuality. He feels that and will internalize this type of interaction and learn to treat others the same way. Additionally, because you are showing your baby the signs for things such as **PLEASE** and **THANK YOU**, he has a way to conceptualize these abstract ideas and use them in his life. Other signs that help introduce the concept of good manners are **HELP, STOP, NO TOUCH, SOFT TOUCH, SHARE**, and **TAKE TURNS**.

You can also help to teach good manners by validating your baby's emotions. When he realizes that you understand he is **SAD** or **HAPPY**, he learns to trust you and feels validated. A child who is secure and validated has a much easier time relating to others and showing them respect. It is never too early to start this process. You should continue to do this for the next several years to create a basis for your child's emotional well-being.

Respecting your baby's pace

If you are fortunate enough to live around other families who sign with their babies, you may be beginning to notice the differences in the children's abilities to sign. Some children may be able to sign fifty to one hundred signs while others only know one or two signs. The consistency with which you sign with your baby makes a lot of difference, but your baby also has his own personal rhythms and reasons for signing. Some children see signing as a tool only to use to get what they need, and others enjoy the process of signing. Your baby could be more interested in conquering some physical milestone at the moment, or he might just be more contemplative before he signs.

Thalia, mom of twins Trinity and Lance, explains. "The twins' abilities are different, their personalities are unique, and their interests are varied. Their differences show up even in their signing. Not only have they chosen to sign at different stages in their development, but the way in which they sign can vary. For instance, Trinity signs **MORE** by touching one finger to the palm of the other hand. Lance signs **MORE** by tapping his fists together and it looks like **SHOES.** I've also noticed that Lance refuses to sign **EAT** because it was one of his first spoken words. Trinity, on the other hand, almost always makes a sign along with the word she's saying out loud. For her, signing and speaking are connected. For Lance it's a tool to use when he can't say a word. Lance always looks for the path of least resistance. Trinity is interested in communication by any form or means."

AHA!

If your baby is doing something that you want him to stop doing, use the sign STOP instead of NO. Babies do not yet understand the multiple meanings of the word NO ("No, do not do that" versus "No, I don't have one of those"). STOP is a more direct way to explain that you want the behavior to stop.

Signs and Activities for Thirteen to Eighteen Months

The sky is the limit when it comes to signing now. You can introduce signs for anything your baby is interested in—and he will be interested in everything. The following suggestions are just that—suggestions. Take your baby's interests and run with them. Sign what you know and learn as you go. Remember, if you don't know the sign for something, you can learn it or use a category sign.

The following section describes some signing activities to try during your daily routine that you and your baby may find entertaining and informative. Specific signs to use are suggested for each activity.

Meal time

More Cereal: Now that your baby has his pincer grasp down and can pick up dry cereal with his fingers, you can play this game with him. Place a piece of dry cereal on his high chair. When he eats it, ask him "Do you want some **MORE**?" Wait until he signs **MORE** to give him another piece. Babies love to play this game and love to be "in charge."

AHA!

Many parents have found that their baby can sit and look at the **Sign Babies ASL Flash Cards** for a long time. Natasha says, "I punched a hole in the top corner of the cards and put them on a ring and string that I attached to Micha's car seat. When we are driving for a long time, she pulls up the string and entertains herself by seeing how many of the cards she can sign. We don't go anywhere without them."

Diaper/Dressing time

Washing Hands: Begin to introduce your baby to the concept of washing his own hands. Because the sign **WASH HANDS** is so descriptive, it helps your baby understand what he needs to do.

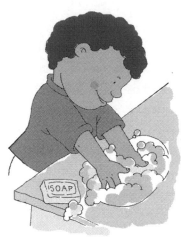

Label Body Parts: During dressing time, label the parts of the body for your baby. Just point to the part of his body and name it. For the most part, the sign for each of the body parts is made by pointing at the body part. This increases his vocabulary and may keep him entertained during dressing.

Activity time

Peek-a-Boo: You can use the structure of the Peek-a-Boo game to show your baby the signs for new words. Hide an object such as a book partially behind your back so your baby can still see it. Then say, "**WHERE** is the **BOOK**? I can't find it. **WHERE** did it go?"

STOP/MORE: One way to reinforce the signs for **STOP** and **MORE** is to play with your baby and then stop and ask him whether he wants more. For example, if you are tickling him, say "**STOP**" and then wait a few seconds and then ask whether he wants **MORE**. This also works for bouncing on the knee or helping him jump up and down. When you are finished playing and do not want to continue the game, say "We are **ALL DONE**." This way he knows it is the end of the game.

TWO CENTS

Parents have so much going on in their daily lives. If you are rushing out the door and you forget to sign **SHOES** when you put your baby's shoes on, don't stress it. The most success in signing comes when you and your baby are not stressed out. Just don't let signing slip for long periods of time or your baby may let his signing slip too.

Animal Signs and Sounds: Babies at this age are very interested in learning about animals. You have probably already introduced some animal signs to your baby, but you will find that now he is even more excited to learn the signs. When you sign and say the name of the animal, add the sound that animal makes. These sounds also allow your baby to practice the basics of speech and help him develop the muscles he needs to speak.

Pet Store/Zoo: Not everyone lives near a farm or close to a zoo or has a lot of pets. A great alternative is the pet store. My son loved a song called "Go to the Zoo," but we live 45 miles from the zoo. Sometimes when we would sing this song and sign the animal signs, he would be desperate to go to the zoo. Instead, we went to the local pet shop and looked at the **FROG**, **RABBIT**, **CAT**, **DOG**, **FISH**, **BIRD**, **MOUSE**, **SNAKE**, **TURTLE**, and **SPIDER** (they had tarantulas). Another alternative is to make a home zoo out of your child's stuffed animals or toys. You can visit this zoo without worrying about strollers, juice cups, or walking long distances. You can even invite friends over to "tour" the zoo with you and your baby, and learn the signs for the animals.

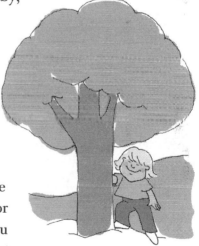

Neighborhood Walk: Take a walk around the neighborhood with your baby. There are so many things for your baby to learn about just outside his door. Some of the wonderful things he can learn about are his **HOUSE**, the **TREE, FLOWER,** and **CLOUDS**. You could comment on the **WIND** or the **SUN**. You could even look at the **BUGS** or listen to the **BIRD**. If a **CAR** goes by or you hear an **AIRPLANE** or a **HELICOPTER**, let him know what these things are by naming and signing them. If a **DOG** barks or a **CAT** walks by, make sure you continue your conversation about these animals as well. As your baby grows, you can even comment on the weather: is it **WARM** or **COLD** or is it **RAINING** or **SNOWING**?

Who Are You?: As we discussed earlier, your baby is gaining a lot of independence. He now knows that he is the **BABY**. Use this understanding to play a game. Say, "Who are you?" and wait for him to sign **BABY**. Then say, "Who are you?" to his dad. He says, "I'm the **DADDY**." Go through all the family members. You can extend this game with a family photo album by asking him "Who is this?" and having him sign **MOM** or **DAD** or **GRANDMA** and so forth.

Hide-and-Seek: A different version of Hide-and-Seek can be played with toys, foods, or other objects you want your baby to learn the signs for. Take plastic food storage containers and hide one object under each of them. It helps to use clear containers until your baby catches on to how to play the game. Ask him, "**WHERE** is the **BALL**? Can you find the **BALL**?" The first time you play the game, you will need to facilitate finding the ball by lifting up the correct container. Say, "Let's look in here." Then, when your baby has found the ball, congratulate him. "You found the **BALL**! **THANK YOU**!" You can also play this game on the high chair with food or in the bathtub with bath toys. As your Hide-and-Seek game becomes more sophisticated, you can add other signs to your sentences such as **FIND**, **PLEASE**, **HELP**, and **LOOK**.

Nursery Rhymes: In addition to songs, classic nursery rhymes are fun and help develop your baby's brain through repetition and rhythm. With nursery rhymes, you are not trying to sign every word. For example, in *Pat-a-Cake*, you might do the following:

Pat-a-cake, pat-a-cake, baker man! (clap hands)
Bake me a **CAKE** as fast as you can!
Put it, and roll it and mark it with a B (roll hands)
And put it in the oven for **BABY** and me!

Or if you are reciting *Little Miss Muffet*, you might want to do the following:

Little Miss Muffet (sign **GIRL**)
SAT on a tuffet
EATING her curds and whey.
Along came a **SPIDER**
Who SAT down beside her
And **FRIGHTENED** Miss Muffet away

Safety time

The Owie Game: In order to reinforce the concept that your baby can tell you where things hurt, play the Owie Game with him. Take one of his stuffed animals (not his favorite one if you think he may cry when it gets "hurt"), and have it accidentally fall down. Say "Oh, Baby that must have **HURT**. Do you need a band aid?" Because children are enthralled with band aids, your baby will love to put a band aid on the pretend owie. Repeat the game and ask other questions such as, "**WHERE** does it **HURT**?" Then pretend you are the stuffed animal and speak in a high voice and say, "It **HURTS** here" and sign where on the animal it hurts. If that place requires another band aid, have your baby put one on. You can extend the game to include stomach aches and teething pain, and give the appropriate medicine. If your child has to go to the doctor or have tests done, this is one way to quiet his fears before the visit. He can be the doctor and help give the shot or take the x-ray. He can tell the doll that it doesn't **HURT**.

Five Little Monkeys Jumping on the Bed: The old rhyme "Five Little Monkeys" is another way to use the sign **HURT**.

Five little **MONKEYS JUMPING** on the **BED**,
One **FELL OFF** and **HURT** his head.
Mama called (**TELEPHONE**) the Doctor and the Doctor said,
"No more **MONKEYS JUMPING** on the **BED**!"

and so on until you get down to one monkey

One little **MONKEY JUMPING** on the **BED**,
He **FELL OFF** and **HURT** his head.
Mama called (**TELEPHONE**) the Doctor and the Doctor said,
"Put those **MONKEYS** straight to **BED**!"

Bath time

Peek-a-Boo in the Bath: You can extend the idea of peek-a-boo to playing in the bathtub by putting a toy under the water and then asking "**WHERE** is the **BOAT**?" Let the toy rise to the surface or let him grab it from under the water.

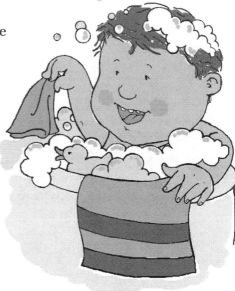

Five Little Ducks: If you have read *Five Little Ducks*, retell this story bath time and use ducks to play out the story. If you don't have six ducks, you can use as many ducks as you have and substitute other objects for the mama duck and some of the baby ducks.

Bedtime

Brush Your Teeth: Sometimes brushing your baby's teeth seems like an impossible task. He doesn't want you to do it and his mouth is so small that the whole thing is difficult. By showing your baby the sign for **BRUSH TEETH**, you can reinforce the idea that brushing teeth is fun. Sing the "Brush Your Teeth" song by Raffi, a popular children's songwriter, or make up your own song to the tune of "Twinkle, Twinkle Little Star." Another way is to make brushing seem fun is to brush the teeth of your baby's dolls and bears. Say, "See how **BEAR BRUSHES** his **TEETH**? **BRUSH** them up and down. Now they are so clean."

Walk or Put the Bear to Bed: A fun ritual to help your baby understand that it's time for bed is to have a **SLEEP** walk in which you say goodnight to your baby's favorite things around the house. When you get to each thing, say **SLEEP** Teddy, **SLEEP** Ball, **SLEEP** Train, etc. By the time you get to your baby's bed, he should be ready to **SLEEP**. You can also put his favorite stuffed animals to **BED**. By putting his bears to **BED**, he sees that everyone is going to bed and prepares himself for sleep.

A Final Note on Helping Your Baby Develop

Signing gives you a way to help your baby understand what he sees in books and in the world around him. Look for your child to translate the knowledge he gains from books into his real life. He may surprise you by relating things from books to his everyday world.

Summary

In this chapter, we discussed:
- ☆ How your baby is developing from thirteen to eighteen months
- ☆ How reading helps his development
- ☆ How your baby's signing abilities will explode
- ☆ How your baby's independence can be influenced by signing
- ☆ Specific activities to use during this period

Bottom Line

Your baby will learn many signs during this time. Expose him to new books and games that give you a chance to sign and expand his vocabulary. Remember that by showing your baby signs, you can help avoid many of the tantrums and struggles that come during this age and later.

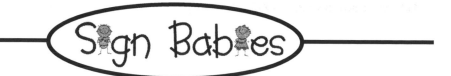
Chapter Six

Nineteen to Twenty-four Months—Look Who's Talking . . . and Signing

For most children, the period from nineteen to twenty-four months is a time to get talking. If your child has not started to talk yet, she will probably do so now. Remember, she has already been communicating with you for months, and possibly even more than a year through her signs. This is not the time to stop signing. You will spend the next several months transitioning from signing and speaking to just speaking. Don't be surprised if your child is still signing at two and a half. Research shows that babies still benefit greatly from signing well into the third year.

In this chapter, we'll take a look at the following:

☆ How your child is developing from nineteen to twenty-four months

☆ Signing and speaking at the same time

☆ Expanding language learning

☆ Continuing good manners

✯ Emotional maturity

✯ Becoming a listener

✯ Specific activities to use during this period

JUST BEGINNING NOW? If you are just beginning to sign with your child, great! Read the previous chapters before you get started. You can expect your child to sign back as quickly as a few days or a week after you begin signing. The signs you start with may be different than if you signed with your child earlier. Start with signs that will motivate your child, such as **FOOD**, **TOYS**, and other signs related to activities she enjoys.

Your Child's Development

At this age, your child is becoming very coordinated and is learning to speak in simple sentences and express her emotions. This is still the time of the Terrible Twos, but signing will lessen the impact on you and your child.

Motor development

Your child is working on the fine motor skills that involve the small muscles in her fingers, hands, and wrists, such as drawing, fitting shapes in a shape sorter, and using a spoon and fork. Her cerebellum, an area of the brain that is important for the timing and coordination of most motor tasks, is also developing and further aids your child's abilities. If your child is not interested in sitting and drawing or writing, don't worry. All forms of fine motor activity–including signing–provide stimulation for her developing brain and motor system.

Don't think that your nineteen-month-old is going to sit and draw or string beads all day. Movement is necessary and extremely important to her sense of well-being. If you confine her too much, she is likely to throw a tantrum. She needs the freedom to move so that she can improve her gross motor skills, the use of the large muscles of the body. When it is safe and appropriate, let her explore her surroundings. It will help her refine her coordination, gain confidence in moving her body through space, release some of her energy, and develop new motor skills such as running, jumping and climbing. Each new motor skill contributes to your child's sense of mastery and her growing feeling of competence.

Language development

The number of words a child uses between nineteen and twenty-four months is related to several factors, such as gender, personality (whether she is outgoing or shy), family size, and so forth. Research indicates that babies who sign with their parents generally speak sooner and have larger vocabularies than their counterparts who do not sign. The average child who does not sign says around 50 words at age two, while babies who sign often speak and/or sign between 150 and 300 words by this age. More importantly, the number of words your child says or signs will increase every month.

The speed at which her vocabulary grows increases exponentially once your child feels comfortable and has a large enough vocabulary to have her basic needs met (somewhere between thirty and sixty words in sign and speech). This can occur as early as fourteen months in babies who sign. Once she reaches this critical mass, she begins adding new words or signs to her vocabulary every day. If your child has not already started to, she will put together two and three word sentences both in sign and words. Often, babies who sign have been creating two and three word sentences in sign and speech for months, but if not, look for this milestone.

As we discussed in previous chapters, research suggests that the amount of language used in conversation with children influences their rate of verbal language development. The more words a child hears while engaged in conversations, the larger her vocabulary will be and the faster it will continue to grow. This is one reason why babies who sign speak sooner and have larger vocabularies than babies who do not–their parents engage them in conversations at an earlier age and more often. Sara was amazed one day when her eighteen-month-old son commented on the weather. "We stepped out of the grocery store, he looked into the sky and said 'Hey Dad, it's a cloudy day.' My jaw dropped; I couldn't believe that he said a full, understandable sentence and even used the correct word tense."

Make sure you take time to listen to your child. If her speech is unclear, try to understand her and use sign to help her express herself. Don't assume you know what she is saying and don't speak for her. By giving her the chance to speak, you give her important practice. You can clarify things by restating what she says and asking her whether you got the correct message.

Cognitive development

At this age, your child learns primarily through hands-on experiences, and her cognitive development is directly related to how many experiences she has. Telling your child about things is not as powerful as allowing her to experience them herself. Giving her a wide variety of sensory, motor and pretend play opportunities is a great way to support her development and doesn't require that you teach her directly. For example, let her mix paint colors to see that yellow and blue make green. Watching this happen is much more instructive for her than hearing you tell her that yellow and blue make green. She has very little capacity to learn just from your words—hands-on experiences can be the best teacher.

Your child now understands that symbols can stand for objects and experiences, a concept called *symbolic representation.*

TWO CENTS

If you suspect that your child is delayed in her speech, talk with your pediatrician. Your pediatrician may want to wait until she is three—when she may be clinically considered speech-delayed—but waiting could cause more problems. If you are uncomfortable waiting, tell your pediatrician. You can also contact your local Regional Center or Early Intervention Program, a state-funded program that helps people with disabilities (consult your state's website), or contact your local school district. By law, every child is entitled to one speech screening. You can also contact the American Speech, Language, and Hearing Association (www.asha.org) to find help.

Because you have been signing with your child, she has already been heavily introduced to this concept. She will begin to extend this under-standing to *symbolic thought* and *pretend play*. She will talk into a toy phone with someone she imagines is on the line or make din-ner out of blocks. Symbolic thought is an important step in learning to read and write and she will soon be able to understand that letters and words represent thoughts.

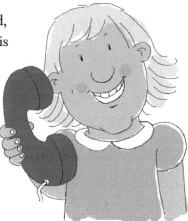

Some children who sign learn the alphabet at this age without a parent's help. This higher cognitive function is a direct result of your child's ability to understand symbolic representation and use symbolic thought. When my son was about sixteen months old, he had a bad cold and we spent the entire day in bed. To break up the day, we watched a Sesame Street video about the alphabet a few times. When he got up that evening, he walked to the refrig-erator and noticed that there were three letters on it. He matter-of-factly said, "C, R, Z." I was shocked because I had never tried teaching him the alpha-bet. Within the next few weeks, he learned the entire alphabet on his own and began reading letters from signs on buildings when we went shopping.

Kim says that all of her children learned the alphabet early on. "My kids used to 'babble' to the alphabet song–a few letters were correct. My older son knew the letters–spoken and signed and most of the sounds–well before he was three years old. It carries through too. My seven-year-old still finger spells words when sounding them out for homework."

Social development

Your child is now developing an awareness of self. She knows that there is not only a "me," but also a "mine." Your child may become very pos-sessive of her toys and even of her parents. This can lead to conflicts, as this is also a time when babies begin to socialize and play in groups. Your child's possessiveness is a way for her to express her independence and autonomy. Understanding this makes understanding her behavior easier. She is not trying to be a brat. She is working out her understanding of self.

Sometimes you can avert problems by explaining. Say, "This is your doll, but can we **SHARE** it with Ella for two minutes. Let's **TAKE TURNS**." When she knows that you know that the doll is hers, she may be more willing to share it. Self-control is still developing at this age. She understands you when you tell her not to take from others, but her lack of self-control may cause her to take it anyway. Self-control comes with time and brain maturation. It is perfectly okay if she has some special toys she does not share with others. You might not want to take these to a play date and make sure you have a special hiding place for them when friends visit.

Helping your child feel that she has some control over her life helps build her self-esteem. When your child has a greater sense that she can make things happen, she has a greater sense of self-competence. Signing gives her a sense that she has a lot of input in her experience. You can enhance this sense of self competence by giving your child simple choices to make. Allow her to choose between two equal things, such as two different shirts or two types of fruit. She wants to have a say in her life. When she feels that she has some control, she is less likely to have temper tantrums.

TWO CENTS

Karen says that her three children put their hands over their eyes when they don't want to know what mom has to say in sign. "It is equal to us holding our hands over our ears so we don't hear, but it's more frustrating because if you yell to an ear-coverer they can still get something. When a child shuts her eyes, there is little you can do except wait for the peek."

Signing and Speaking at the Same Time

During your child's transition to spoken language, you will find that she continues to sign words that she is able to speak. She does this for several reasons. First, she has not mastered pronunciation and intonation yet, and signing helps her get her message out. If she notices that you don't understand her, she will use a sign for clarification. Second, she might use a sign as a way to underscore the importance of the word. Many mothers report that long after their children can speak clearly—even sometimes as late as four or five years old—their children will sign and say **PLEASE** whenever they really want something. Signing seems to function like an exclamation point for these children, giving them a way to add emphasis. Finally, your child might just enjoy the movement and action involved in signing. Some parents and children find signing so enjoyable that they go on to learn more about ASL.

As your child confronts difficult situations, she can lose the ability to communicate when she gets frustrated. Signing can also help her in this area, because the motor control needed to make signs requires less from your child than the motor control needed to form words. Adults often lose their ability to communicate when they are frustrated. How many times have you felt speechless when something has happened? But we generally recover quickly. Your child lacks the experience to know what to do when she is at a loss for words. In times like these, keep your cool and remind your child to "Use your hands (**SIGN**)" so that she remembers she can speak with sign until her ability to talk returns. Children who do not have sign language to fall back on often resort to screaming or hitting to get their point across. You will see less of this behavior if your child has a back-up language system. For this reason alone, many preschools have begun teaching signs to children not previously exposed to child sign language so that they will have a way to communicate when they are frustrated.

Whatever your child's reason for signing, if she knows how to say the word, don't worry. She will not be hampered in her transition to spoken language by signing. The bridge you have given her remains there for her to use whenever she needs it.

Expanding Language Learning

Continue to expand your child's language experience through *stretch talk* (adding to what your child says). When your child initiates a conversation by signing something to you that you did not ask her about, make sure that you extend the conversation by asking her more questions or providing her with more information.

If she says or signs **KITTY**, say "Yes, that **KITTY** is **SOFT** and **LITTLE**." If your child comments on the fact that **DADDY** is **EATING**, you can extend the comment to a conversation by asking questions such as "**WHAT** is **DADDY EATING**?" Give your child time to answer back. If she doesn't answer back, try asking her such silly questions as "Is he **EATING BEARS** or **SHOES**?" Often silly questions prompt a response. When she tells you what he is eating, confirm it for her. "Yes, **DADDY** is **EATING APPLES**."

Extend the language learning to a game. When you play hide-and-seek, add a linguistic element to your game. Think out loud about where your child might be hiding to introduce or reinforce vocabulary. Say "**WHERE** is Alexa?" and then add, "Maybe she is in the refrigerator next to the **MILK**?" The nonsense in this sentence is funny to your child, but helps her learn more complex words. She knows that there is a place where the milk goes, but she might not know that it is called the refrigerator. She is listening to you because she wants to be found, so you have a captive audience. Or play a simplified version of Simon Says. Say, "Show me your nose. Show me your toes."

Finally, children at this age are beginning to enjoy language for language's sake. They begin to understand the words to rhymes and enjoy the sound of the rhymes. Now that your child knows the rhymes to the songs you sing often, change the words and signs a bit and see what she does. You can also introduce her to nonsensical books. She will begin to understand the irony in these books. Or make up funny names for things your child knows the name for. Playing with language helps children understand the rhythm of language.

Continuing the Good Manners

You can continue to model basic good manners by signing and saying **PLEASE, THANK YOU, SORRY, TAKE TURNS**, and **SHARE**. The best way to teach manners is to lead by example. Use good manners and use polite language: "**DADDY, PLEASE** pass me the carrots. Oh **THANK YOU**." If you exaggerate the **PLEASE** and **THANK YOU**, it makes the words more interesting to your child. You can even extend the good manners lesson to play time. Have a tea party with your child's dolls or stuffed animals and use the words for good manners. Allow your child to interact and ask her dolls to **PLEASE** pass the **COOKIES**.

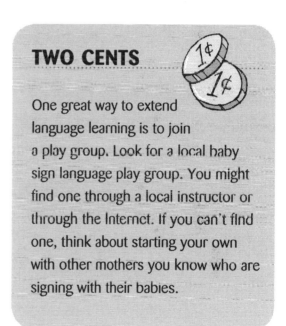

TWO CENTS

One great way to extend language learning is to join a play group. Look for a local baby sign language play group. You might find one through a local instructor or through the Internet. If you can't find one, think about starting your own with other mothers you know who are signing with their babies.

Praise your child when she uses any of the signs or words for good manners. She will be encouraged to continue using her good manners if she is rewarded emotionally each time. This is the age when you will start arranging play dates with other moms. If their children are also signing, look to see whether the children sign together. Often, when your child needs to ask for something, she will sign **PLEASE** to her playmates, even if she won't sign **PLEASE** with you.

Make sure that in addition to using the words and the signs, your voice and face match the word and the feeling you are trying to convey. For example,

TWO CENTS

One of the best things about teaching your child manners with sign is that when she gets older, you can remind her to use her manners from across the room. When Grandma gives her a present for her third birthday, you can sign "**SAY THANK YOU**" to remind her to use her good manners.

if you say **SORRY** to your child, make sure your face looks sorry, and your voice sounds sorry. Exaggeration helps. If you have done something that requires an apology, make sure your child sees you sign **SORRY**. You can also teach your child to use this sign when she has done something that needs an apology.

Reading books together on good manners also helps your child see that manners were not just your idea. Especially when children get past age two, books like these are very effective. One good book is *It's Neat to Eat at the Table* by Lindy Bartell. The story is about Perry and Penny Pig, and how they learn to use good manners.

Emotional Maturity

From the day your child was born, you have probably dreaded the day when she would throw tantrums. Because you sign with your child, you might have found that you have not experienced as many tantrums as parents who have children of the same age. Most tantrums occur because a child feels little sense of control, cannot get her point across, or cannot get her needs met. Signing has helped your child in this area because she has a sense of control over her environment, she has an ability to get her point across, and she can get her needs met.

You will also begin to notice that your child's range of emotions is growing. She is now showing you signs of pride, frustration, timidity, and also exhilaration and fierce independence. As she learns the gamut of emotions, you will need to deal with them. Sometimes, this leads to conflict and issues. Signing can help you give names to the emotions and help her learn to deal with them. You can show her the signs and names for emotions such as **ANGRY**, **HAPPY**, **SAD**, **PROUD**, and **SHY** so that she can express what she is feeling to you. This will help her cope with the emotions, and will help her express them to you. If she has acted improperly, you can validate and acknowledge her feelings while letting her know that her actions were not acceptable.

Always remember *not* to mistake your child's verbal and signing abilities for emotional maturity. She might be able to talk or sign to you words that are well beyond her age, but she is still very young and emotionally immature. Allow her to be a child and give her a chance to learn about her new emotions. If you can, avoid situations that cause problems. For example, if you know she gets edgy when she is hungry, carry snacks. Or, if she is exhausted in the grocery store and heading for a meltdown, leave the cart with the manager and take her home and put her to bed. Sometimes, you have to step in and be the parent and help her before she has a meltdown. Sometimes this means sacrificing your own schedule for her benefit.

TWO CENTS

Most children in the United States don't get enough sleep. Your child should still be getting twelve to thirteen hours of sleep with naps and nighttime sleep. Sleep will help your child have a balanced life and better experiences when she is awake.

Becoming a Good Listener

Listening is a skill that your child develops with practice. It will help your child in social interactions, learning experiences, and when she needs to gain information. As she gets older, listening will become essential to her educational experiences. Now is a good time to start helping her develop listening skills. Just as you have been doing since you started signing with your child, get your child's attention by calling her name or touching her. Then speak slowly to her and sign to her. Use parallel talk and sign (tell her what she is doing) or self-talk and sign (tell her what you are doing) to focus your child's attention.

Here are some other ideas:

☆ Play games that require your child to listen to your directions. Ask her to "**LOOK** for the **BALL**" or "**HIDE** your **BEAR** under the **BLANKET**." Your child must listen to you to complete these tasks.

☆ Change the tone of your voice for different characters when you read books or recite rhymes, chants, and fingerplays. This will help her listen more closely to your story.

☆ Point out the sounds around your child. If a dog barks, say, "Do you **HEAR** that? It is a **DOG** barking."

☆ Spend time listening to music. Introduce your child to different types of music, such as classical, jazz, country, folk, popular, and children's music. You can even make some instruments such as rhythm sticks, shakers, cymbals, and drums out of household items.

☆ Sing songs to your child. She might even join in at this age. Simple songs that repeat a "surprise" element are the best. *Old MacDonald* and *B-I-N-G-O* work well because your child has to listen for the animal or for the letter that is missing in the next verse. These songs might be getting old for you, but she will love them for years to come.

It takes a lot of control and practice for your child to listen. Practice now will reap rewards later. But be patient and always remember that she is only a baby.

Signs and Activities for Nineteen to Twenty-Four Months

You and your child have been signing for quite a while now, and you have an amazing repertoire of signs under your belt. You may not need to add more signs to communicate. Instead, expand the situations in which you use signs to give your child more language experiences. If you and your child want to learn more signs, now is a great time to learn descriptor signs for colors and size so that your child can better describe the world around her. Also, because she wants to express her independence, now is a great time to get her involved in household activities and let her "help" you.

The following section describes some signing activities that you and your baby may find entertaining and informative. Specific signs to use are suggested for each activity.

So big, so small

Now is a good time to help your child learn how to describe her world. An easy way for her to start is to play "So Big, So Small." While you are playing with your child, gather several things together that are different in size—some big and some small. To introduce the game, say "Oh, this **BEAR** is so **BIG** and this **CAR** is so **SMALL**!" Repeat this a few times with different toys. Just keep it fun and exciting. Extend this game to your daily activities by explaining that things are big or small.

If you want to introduce colors or other descriptors to your child, you can change this activity to point out the colors of different objects. Gather several objects with colors together. Then say, "This **FROG** is **GREEN** and this **CAR** is **RED**." Continue the game by adding different objects and describing things in your daily activities. "These **APPLES** are **GREEN** and this **BANANA** is **YELLOW**."

TWO CENTS

It's a mistake to do everything for your child, because you are preparing her for adulthood. Enlist her to **CLEAN UP** toys with you. Ask her to **HELP** you make her bed. If she can't pull the sheets up or tuck the blanket in, make it her job to put on the **PILLOW**. Then say "**THANK YOU** so much for your **HELP**. I couldn't have done it without you. You put the **PILLOW** in just the right place." You build her sense of accomplishment and teach her to work together with others.

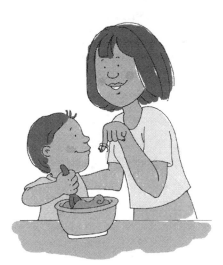

You don't need to worry about quizzing your child. She is not in school yet and doesn't need a test. Just play "So Big, So Small" and continue the game by describing things she interacts with. She will learn descriptors naturally.

Helping around the house

Your child wants to help you do things. She feels big enough to participate more actively in daily activities. Find ways to incorporate her and ask her for her **HELP**. By inviting her to participate, you are teaching her social skills, language skills, intellectual concepts, and responsibility. You are also reinforcing the idea that activities have a beginning, middle, and an end. You also teach her that families work together.

When you are making dinner, create an area where she can **COOK** with you. Empty out a cupboard or create a special zone where she can pretend to prepare dinner. While you are making dinner, she may become engrossed in her own meal preparations and may be content to play without your interaction.

If your child needs to interact with you while she is preparing her "meal," take advantage of this time to ask her questions and sign with her. You can also *parallel talk* and sign (tell her what she is doing) or *self-talk* and sign (tell her what you are doing) to comment on what she is doing in both sign and words. If you change out items in the cupboard, ask her "**WHAT** is that?" and then explain to her what it is and how it is used.

Walk and stop

To teach your child to have control and listen to your commands, you can use this simple game. It is called "Walk and Stop." It is a simplified, musical version of Simon Says. Using the tune of "Twinkle, Twinkle Little Star," sing and sign the following:

AHA!

Your child may only be capable of independent play for thirty to sixty seconds. Instead of getting frustrated, intermittently interact with her by asking questions or participating in her play. You are helping her learn how to play independently, but that skill might not be well-developed until your child is three or four years old.

WALK and **WALK** and **WALK** and **STOP**
WALK and **WALK** and **WALK** and **STOP**
WALK and **WALK** and **WALK** and **STOP**
WALK and **WALK** and **WALK** and **STOP**
WALK and **WALK** and **WALK** and **STOP**
WALK and **WALK** and **WALK** and **STOP**

Your child should **WALK** until you say **STOP**. Pause when you say **STOP** to give your child some time to process the command. Even though this seems simple for you, it is a very complex skill for your child to master. It requires impulse control, motor control, and cognitive control. Once she has mastered this game, change it a bit by first changing the action to **JUMP** or **DANCE** or **SWING**. Then, once she has mastered the change, add another dimension. Change when the **STOP** command is given.

WALK and **STOP** and **WALK** and **STOP**
WALK and **WALK** and **STOP** and **WALK**
STOP and **WALK** and **WALK** and **STOP**
WALK and **WALK** and **WALK** and **STOP**
STOP and **WALK** and **WALK** and **STOP**
WALK and **WALK** and **WALK** and **STOP**

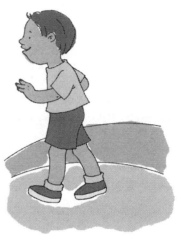

Once again, pause when you say **STOP** to give your child time to process the command. By playing this simple game, you are teaching your child to coordinate the skills necessary for learning to listen to what you say. Children at this age don't necessarily blatantly disobey their parents. Sometimes they just cannot process all the information and respond to the command.

Silly mommy

One of the best things you can do for your child is to teach her that making mistakes is a part of growing up, and that it is safe to make mistakes as she is learning. You are becoming well aware that your child will do something the wrong way tons of times before she gets it right—such as getting her shoes on the right feet or keeping her spoon on the table.

Barbara explains how she taught her daughter how to be okay with making mistakes. "When my daughter Shira began to show an interest in dressing herself, I introduced the signs for **MISTAKE/WRONG**, **SILLY**, and **RIGHT/CORRECT**. When I was dressing Shira or sometimes myself, I would put the shoes on the wrong feet or some other article of clothing on incorrectly. I would then laugh and say '**WRONG ME. SILLY MOMMY**.' Then I would put the shoes or clothing on correctly and say '**RIGHT**,' with a very proud look on my face. When Shira began to dress herself, she naturally made mistakes, and she was able to say '**WRONG ME**' and would try again until she got it '**RIGHT**.' I truly believe this decreased her frustration in taking on a new developmental task by having the language to talk about what was happening." Try this as a safe way to introduce the concept that it is okay to make a mistake, and it is good to fix things that go wrong. You can also say "Let's try it **AGAIN**." Your child will feel safe to come to you when she has done something wrong, and ask you for help or do it herself until she gets it right.

Naming emotions

As your child matures into her emotions, giving her different feelings a name as a way to express them is very useful. Modeling and labeling with words and signs are the best way to help your child identify emotions. If you are playing and everyone is laughing and being silly, you can take that opportunity to say, "I feel **SILLY** and I feel **HAPPY**." That way, your child learns the words for how she is feeling. You can also use books and songs to teach your child what emotions are. One book that helps teach moods and emotions is *Today I Feel Silly and Other Moods That Make My Day* by Jamie Lee Curtis. Another is *Curious George's Are You Curious?* by H. A. Rey.

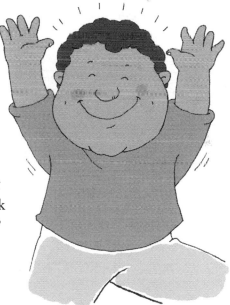

If you have puppets or stuffed animals, play out emotions with them to model for your child what different emotions look like. Or you can play the "Feeling Game." First you model what feelings look like and then you say "Show me what **SAD** looks like. Show me what you look like when you're **HAPPY**."

Around town

Turn your experiences around town into learning experiences. If you have a fun excursion such as a trip to the zoo, make sure you name all the **ANIMALS** for your child. Even if you just have regular chores and trips, you can turn them into opportunities to learn language. For example, a trip to the grocery store can introduce concepts and words to your child. Tell your child about what you are seeing and ask her for help. Have her tell you what the foods are and ask her to watch out for certain items.

Say, "**WHERE** are the **APPLES**?" Have her help you put the apples in the bag. Ask her "Do we need **MORE APPLES**?" Have her hold things that are safe for her to hold. Remember that for a trip to be successful, you should only go when your child is rested and spend only a short time. As adults, we want to get everything done at once, but children can't take that much mental stimulus and need their naps. Don't sacrifice your child's well-being to get that last errand in.

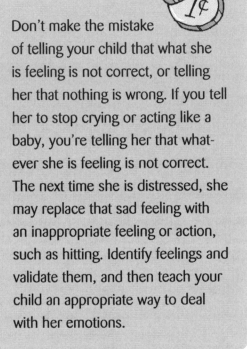

TWO CENTS

Don't make the mistake of telling your child that what she is feeling is not correct, or telling her that nothing is wrong. If you tell her to stop crying or acting like a baby, you're telling her that whatever she is feeling is not correct. The next time she is distressed, she may replace that sad feeling with an inappropriate feeling or action, such as hitting. Identify feelings and validate them, and then teach your child an appropriate way to deal with her emotions.

Fun at bedtime

A classic song that is fun to sign at bedtime is "Ten in the Bed."

There were ten in the **BED**
And the little one said,
"Roll over! Roll over!"

So they all rolled over and one **FELL OUT (FALL DOWN)** . . .

There were nine in the **BED**
And the little one said,
"Roll over! Roll over!"
So they all rolled over and one **FELL OUT (FALL DOWN)** . . .

There were eight in the **BED**
And the little one said,
"Roll over! Roll over!"
So they all rolled over and one **FELL OUT (FALL DOWN)** . . .

Down to the last line

There was one in the **BED**
And the little one said,
"GOOD NIGHT!"

A Final Note on Helping Your Child's Vocabulary

You and your child have now been partners in signing for a long time. Expanding the situations in which your child can sign will help expand her understanding of language. Using parallel talk and stretch talk to add words to her conversations will help your child have a larger vocabulary.

One way to empower your child is to let her show you how much she

TWO CENTS

Your child's short-term memory is quite good, but she does not have a good sense of time. She can name the animals that she saw at the zoo, but can't remember when she went. Even though she might not remember the exact time and details of your excursions, these experiences help her construct ideas about the world around her.

AHA!

A great online resource for early learning songs comes from BBC Radio, which hosts "Listen and Play," a twenty-eight-part audio resource for preschool children emphasizing the development of early literacy skills. Each program includes familiar songs, rhymes, stories, and sound discrimination games to develop children's phonological awareness and confidence with spoken language. The songs and games in this program can easily be adapted for use with your baby to enhance your experience in signing (see www.bbc.co.uk/ schoolradio/ earlylearning/ listenandplay.shtml).

does know. Jessica's son, Dallin, was not talking for a long time. However, he was very proud that he could sign every one of the one hundred signs in the *Sign Babies ASL Flash Cards.* He would bring the photo album, where she stored the cards, to her lap and sign every sign. He beamed with joy. Soon after, he learned all the signs and his confidence got stronger. He began to speak with the signs. His vocabulary has been steadily growing ever since.

Summary

In this chapter, we discussed:

☆ How your child is developing from nineteen to twenty-four months

☆ Signing and speaking at the same time

☆ Expanding language learning

☆ Continuing good manners

☆ Emotional maturity

☆ Becoming a listener

☆ Specific activities to use during this period

Bottom Line

Now is a good time to expand your child's vocabulary by introducing descriptor signs and giving her words and signs for the things she is feeling and experiencing. Using parallel talk and stretch talk to add signs and words is a great way to help expand her vocabulary.

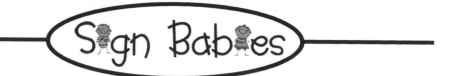

Chapter Seven

Two Years and Beyond— What Can I Do with Signing Now?

You and your child have come a long way since you began your signing journey. Now that you are embarking on the third year of your child's life, you might be wondering whether signing will continue to play an important role. Research shows that children can benefit from signing even in their preschool and kindergarten years. Some schools are even adding signing to their curriculums to help reading and classroom management. Most parents and children stop signing somewhere before children are three, but you might be surprised by how long signing can be of use to you.

In this chapter, we look at the following:
☆ How your child is developing at two years
☆ The long-term effects of signing
☆ Continuing to sign

☆ Losing signs
☆ Encouraging speech

JUST BEGINNING NOW? If you are just starting to sign with your child, read all of the previous chapters before you begin signing with him. You can expect him to sign as quickly as a few days or a week after you begin signing.

Your Child's Development

Your child is quite independent now, and is capable of letting you know what he needs. He is still developing his fine motor skills and will greatly improve his language skills over the next year. He is also working out the rules of social interaction. Signing will help him develop in all of these areas while giving him a way to communicate when he is frustrated or can't yet say the words.

AHA!

Potty training is something you will face soon if you haven't started already. Remember to use your signs to help your child be successful. Signs such as **WET**, **DIRTY**, **CHANGE**, and **POTTY** can help him signal to you that he either needs to go or has missed the opportunity. He might be embarrassed to tell you in words but will tell you with signs.

Motor development

As your child grows, his brain continues to develop and his fine motor skills improve. Practicing skills reinforces the growth of brain cells and the developing connections between them. Your child will become better at tasks such as dressing, feeding himself, getting a drink, washing his hands, stringing beads, using a paint brush, cutting with scissors, drawing with crayons, throwing and kicking a ball, hopping on one foot, pedaling a tricycle, and climbing up and down a small slide. He will also be very proficient at signing by now.

You might notice that he develops a preference for one hand or the other.

Typically, a child switches back and forth several times before settling on a preferred hand. He might even switch which hand he signs with. Don't worry. He is just mastering his motor skills. His dominant hand will become apparent around age four.

Language development

By the time he is three, your child will have a vocabulary of at least 900 words and use three- to five-word sentences. However, prepare yourself. Because you signed with your child, his vocabulary might be twice as large as the average child's vocabulary. He will be able to express himself very well.

If you have been using multiple spoken languages in your house in addition to signing, you will begin to see that your child can differentiate the two languages. As discussed in earlier chapters, your child is capable of learning two or more languages simultaneously as long as he is in a consistent, caring relationship with someone who speaks each language. Your child needs a reliable language partner when speaking and learning each particular language, so if you speak English and your spouse speaks Spanish, keep it that way.

If you have been using English and sign only, your child can also differentiate the two and will know who to sign with and who to speak with. Lauri teaches baby sign language in Canada and says, "In my Sign & Say classes in Winnipeg, Max will sign because he sees everyone else using signs. But if we are with extended family, or others, he'll talk. At his day care, he would not use sign until the day care provider used a sign with him once. He then started regularly signing to him. Like other bilingual children, they quickly learn who uses what language and can switch effortlessly."

If you are bilingual but have not spoken to your child in the other language, now is a great time to use his signing abilities to introduce the other language. Children become fascinated with language for language's sake between two and four years old. Begin speaking the other language and use the same signs as you used when speaking English. Thalia says, "I speak

Spanish fluently, but have found it nearly impossible to speak to my twins in Spanish consistently. Recently, I've discovered that sign language is an excellent bridge to the two languages. I can say *perro* as I sign **DOG** and my little girl signs **DOG** back to me. Then I ask her to sign *perro* and sure enough, she begins slapping her leg. I'm excited by the possibility of using sign to bridge English and Spanish. Perhaps I haven't failed at teaching Spanish just yet!"

Cognitive development

Crazy as it may sound, some parents consider putting their children in school as soon as they turn two. They feel that this gives their children a competitive edge later in their educational experiences. Clearly, you want to do the best you can to create a positive, supportive learning environment for your child—one that optimizes brain growth and all areas of development. But a structured school environment is not necessary to do that. Research shows that just playing is the best thing for your child. He is now learning to incorporate his real-life experiences into pretend play. This is his way of figuring out the world around him. The best things you can do are:

- ☆ Help him create imaginative games and think of new ways to use toys. Blocks can be food or animals in a pretend zoo.
- ☆ Give him time to play by himself. Playing alone gives him a chance to process and understand what he has been doing and learning all day.
- ☆ When you read together, ask questions about the book to include him in the story and to make sure he understands.
- ☆ Point to the words when you are reading to help him understand the process of reading. Encourage him to sign and say the words he knows.
- ☆ Provide materials to scribble, draw, or pretend to write.

If you are worried that your child won't love books and music unless he has classes and attends structured story time, relax. Just expose him to books and music and let him watch you use them in your life. Your example is very important. If you must place your child in day care, look for a day care provider that signs with the children or someone willing to learn how to sign a few signs. This will make the transition easier for your child and help continue the process of learning.

Your child will ask the question "Why" more frequently. He is naturally curious and wants to learn. Instead of being frustrated when he asks why for the tenth time, see it as an opportunity to engage his brain. Sometimes you can even reverse the question session and ask him why.

Social development

Two-year-olds are highly involved in their emerging sense of self and cannot fully understand another child's perspective. Additionally, your child is still developing control over his emotions. He may show outbursts of anger and frustration at the same time he is learning to deal with emotions such as shame, wariness, anxiety, fear, pleasure, pride, and joy. Children who have ways to express their emotions with language have an easier time navigating the sometimes-explosive emotions of toddlerhood. You can help your child by identifying his emotions and giving him words and signs to express them. If he is happy, say "I can see that you are **HAPPY**. You have such a big smile on your face."

Or, if he has hit another child, say "I can see you are **ANGRY**. It is okay to be **ANGRY**, but we don't **HIT**. Use your words instead." Always acknowledge your child's feelings and then offer

AHA!

Don't let TV stand in for you as your child's teacher. The average child watches three to four hours a day, despite recommendations from the American Academy of Pediatrics that children should watch no more than an hour or two a day, and that children under two should watch no television at all. TV watching comes at the expense of parental interaction and other activities such as playing. Limit the time your child watches to two thirty-minute sessions. Carefully select the programs you allow your child to watch, choosing educational programs without commercials. Interact with your child while he is watching so that he does not zone out.

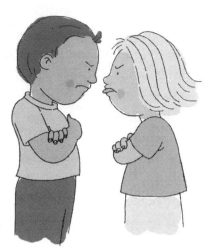

him concrete consequences for negative behaviors and stick to them. You can also use coping mechanisms such as taking deep breaths, sitting in a comfy chair, looking at a happy book, or getting a glass of water. Now is a critical time to teach your child how to deal with emotions in addition to validating them. Things won't change overnight, but as you give him words to express his emotions, he will gain greater self-control.

The Long-Term Effects of Signing

The positive effects of signing with babies outlast the signs themselves. In fact, signing can have such a positive effect on your child's learning experiences that the effects have been measured through age twelve. Research funded by the National Institutes of Health has shown that at age four, children who signed as babies are linguistically advanced when compared to children who did not sign. These same children were tested at ages eight and twelve and were found to have a higher IQ than their counterparts who did not sign—an average of twelve points higher.

Barbara is a speech-language pathologist who has three-year-old twins. Because of her training, she was well aware of how her children were developing linguistically and knew that babies who sign make sentences up to six months earlier and often are far ahead of other children in their linguistic development. Her children's language skills are at least one to one and a half years above their age.

WOW

Sue says, "My two-year-old Erika has phased out all of her signs, except for **SORRY**, which she will do really fast in a big circle around her stomach when I ask her to say **SORRY**."

By eighteen months they were using at least three to five words together; by two years they were speaking in five- to seven-word sentences with various types of grammatical forms. Barbara always encourages parents to sign, even though their child may not sign back, because "good results and improved language skills can still occur. And I encourage them to continue signing after their kids start to talk. I'm sure that is what helped my kids learn their colors and shapes so early."

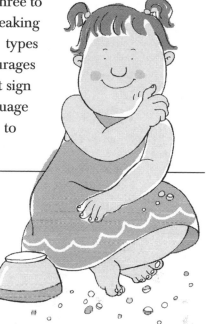

Because babies who sign start communicating earlier, they are exposed to more language opportunities. This increases their vocabulary and allows them to express complex thoughts earlier. Babies who sign can express abstract concepts such as **SAD** or **HUNGRY** that babies of the same age might not be able to express. Babies who cannot sign have to wait until they develop the complex dance of muscles required to say words.

Your child can explain that she dumped the **CEREAL**.

Barbara shared the following experience, "My kids understood many more signs than they used as infants and young toddlers. The proof is in their current level of language skills. I signed more to them than they signed to me, but they still got great benefits from it. Recently, on the way to preschool, my three-year-old daughter asked me 'What makes the wind? Do the trees make the wind?' So I said something like 'No, the clouds move and that make the wind.' She replied with 'So, the clouds make the wind, the wind moves the leaves, and the leaves fall off the trees' while looking out the window at the leaves. I was amazed at the sequential connection that she had made!"

WOW

Jen says, "A few months ago I had to be gone overnight and my two-year-old daughter stayed with her grandma. When she woke up she cried and asked for me. Grandma expressed her sympathy. My daughter responded, 'I supposed to be with my mama so I had to cry! ' Then today she was getting her hair cut and the lady asked her how old she was and she responded, 'I'm gonna be three in March.' I just about fell out of the chair! I was expecting her to say two because she is only two and a half."

When babies who sign begin to speak, they often have better pronunciation and larger vocabularies. This might be because their parents speak face-to-face with them more often. When you speak with your child face-to-face, he can hear your voice and see your mouth. You will begin to notice that your child's pronunciation far outpaces that of many of his counterparts. He will be better understood by adults, which will increase his self-esteem. Also, your child will not be as timid about starting or participating in conversations because he has been initiating conversations with you for a long time now. When my son signed **MOON** when we were outside one night, I said "Yes, that is the **MOON**. Do you see the **STARS**?" He started it and I extended it. Later, he was not afraid to start a conversation and discuss even in-depth topics because he had this early experience in conversing with adults.

Continuing to Sign

Because your child can now communicate with both speech and sign, signing takes on a different dimension. It is not *just* for communicating basic needs anymore. You can show your child signs for things he is interested in or needs help with. You can show him signs for multisyllabic words that are hard to pronounce. He will never stop using his hands in some way when he speaks. Even adults use their hands to indicate things such as size, to emphasize words, or to communicate complete thoughts. For example, you might see your friend at a distance and want to tell him to call you so you sign **TELEPHONE** so that he knows to call you.

If you have another baby, signing gives your child something that he can show his baby brother and a reason to keep signing. Put him "in charge" of signing with his brother. Being in charge gives him a way to bond with his brother and gives him a sense of his independence and importance in the family. Signing with the second child is a way for you to help decrease sibling tensions and increase communication bonds. Just as you started with only a few signs with your first child, do the same with his siblings.

Some children become enthralled with the idea of learning American Sign Language for the sake of learning a language. Often, this interest starts somewhere between three and five years old. If your child becomes interested in learning ASL, take the opportunity to introduce him to more signs and especially more of the language structure. Take him to community classes if you have them, or try some of the DVDs made specifically for older children. Appendix C lists recommended DVDs you can use.

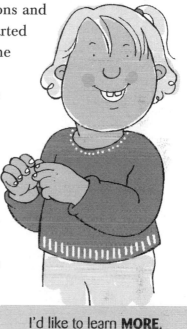

I'd like to learn **MORE**.

Using Signs to Introduce the Alphabet

Many parents who sign with their children take advantage of this skill to introduce their children to the alphabet. The alphabet is a system of symbols, just like signing, so children make the leap from the hand movement to the sound to the alphabet symbol easily. This is a good time to show your child the manual alphabet (the signs for all the letters) while you are introducing

AHA

Holly says, "My son liked to visit with the fish in his sister's class at day care. He would sign FISH almost as soon as he saw the day care building. When I took him to his class he would be so distraught, waving his hands and screaming. I thought it was because I was leaving him. Then I noticed that while I was still there, he was signing FISH while screaming. The day I realized he was signing FISH, I took him to the pet store and we picked out a beautiful beta and donated the fish to his classroom. Now he willingly goes to class, takes off his coat and his first sign is FISH. When we leave, he signs I LOVE YOU to the fish, blows it a kiss and says bye-bye. What an ah-ha moment for me!"

the sounds for the letters and the symbols (written on the page). Singing the alphabet song is a good way to practice.

If you have not finger spelled words with your child, now is a good time to do that as well. Start with simple three-letter words and work from there. As Lauri found out, there are other advantages to teaching your child the alphabet through his hands. "I've seen Megan, who is three, get stuck on the **LMNO** part of the alphabet (speaking) and then look to my hands for the signs, and then use that to help her remember the English. In English, the **LMNO** seems like one complicated word. The signs separate them into four letters more visually, and seem to help her remember."

As your child progresses and learns more finger spelling, don't be surprised if he asks you to "spell it in your hand." When Alex was three, he came to his mother Nina and asked her how to spell the word **DAD**. "I told him quickly, thinking that he was too young to understand. He then looked at me and said, 'Mom, spell it in your hand.' We had been doing a little bit of finger spelling, but nothing significant. I guess he got the concept and wanted to know how to spell that word. I spelled it for him and he practiced it for a few minutes. Often, he would ask me to 'spell it in your hand' when he wanted to know how a word was spelled."

Sometimes, your child will even learn to spell words without you knowing it. Barbara says that shortly before her daughter Shira turned two, they were "driving through a small beach town, when we came to a four-way stop. From the back seat Shira says and finger spells, '**S T O P**. That spells **STOP**!' I had no idea she could read the sign, much less spell it!"

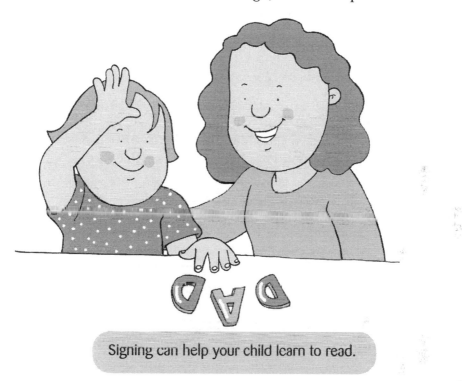

Signing can help your child learn to read.

Losing Signs

You and your child have learned a lot of signs. The process has brought you closer together and given you a chance to bond with your child. You might be surprised by how sad you are when your child begins the process of using only speech without signs. Signing has given both of you comfort and peace. But like all things with your child, he is growing in stages and is changing every day. Children stop signing when they feel confident in their ability to get their point across. If your child has advanced so much in his speech that he feels comfortable with speaking only, be happy! You have met your goal— to bridge the communication gap until your child could speak.

Generally, children stop signing in stages. First, he will sign and say words that he knows how to say. Then, gradually, the signs will drop off and the words will take over. He will keep a few signs for emphasis or clarification of words he still cannot pronounce. Then, finally, words will take over completely and he will stop signing unless there is a reason to sign, like a new child or a deaf family member.

Even when your child has a well-developed vocabulary, he might hold on to a few signs that help him communicate better. For example, he might continue to sign **POTTY** so that he can secretly let you know that he has to go potty. Parents report that this is one sign they kept for years after their babies stopped signing as a simple way to ask their child without embarrassing him. Another sign that hangs around for a long time is **HELP**. You can ask your child whether he needs help without saying anything. Sometimes independent souls don't want anyone to know that they need help, and this sign gives your child a way to communicate without becoming embarrassed. You also might need to tell your child to **STOP** what he is doing without embarrassing him.

ONLINE

The online radio show Babies and Moms: Birth and Beyond (www.babiesandmomsradio.com) has some excellent podcasts about signing with older children—even children who did not sign as babies. Check them out.

Many children enjoy signing **PLEASE** and **THANK YOU** as a way to show that they really mean what they are saying. Some mothers have found that **WAIT** serves them well when they are in a place such as church or synagogue where their kids need to be quiet and sit still. Probably the most prevalent sign that continues with families who have signed with one or more children is **I LOVE YOU**. For obvious reasons, this sign is the longest-lasting sign. Parents can show their children who are performing in the school pageant that they love and support them. Kids can show their parents that they love them as they are driving off to Grandma's house for a sleepover.

Signing also comes in handy when you need to communicate with your mouth full or when you want to communicate when you are on the phone.

Encouraging Speech

Your goal from the beginning of this journey has been to help your hearing child learn to use language and to speak. Now that he is well on his way to yapping your ear off and running up huge cell phone bills, there are a few things you can do to ensure the success of his transition to speech.

1. Do not speak "baby talk" to your child. He is capable of learning cut, scrape, and bruise instead of using boo-boo for every injury. In the long run, when you avoid "baby talk," you are helping him extend his vocabulary and increase his ability to express his needs, wants, and desires.

2. Always respond to your child's attempts to communicate. Don't ignore your child even if you are involved in something else. Acknowledge him and ask him to **WAIT** for his turn. This is a difficult concept for him to learn because he is now brimming with desire to communicate. But ignoring him sends the wrong message.

3. Continue to use the speaking skills

AHA!

If you want to teach your child ASL, now is a good time to introduce more signs, finger spelling, and ASL grammar. Around three years old, your child may become interested in languages not just for communicating, but for the idea of learning a new language. You can capitalize on this and introduce him to more ASL. If you are not fluent in ASL, try some videos such as **Sign-a-Lot** or **Signing Time** to add more signs. Or check your library for other ASL DVDs. There are DVDs that teach how to sign songs, poems, and stories.

you learned when you began signing with your child, including looking directly at your child when you speak (unless driving), speaking slowly and clearly, and using complete sentences.

4. Make sure that your requests to your child are simple and direct. Do not ask him three questions at once. Ask one question, wait for his to reply, and then ask him another question. This allows your child to process each request and respond. Or give him one task such as "Pick up your toy" before you give him another task.

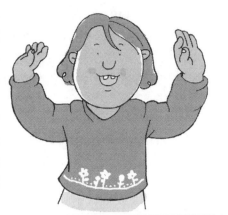

Some children sign **ALL DONE** by raising hands high.

5. Continue to read with your child. Reading exposes him to language he might not hear in daily conversation. Reading with your child also exposes him to letters and words and provides one of the first steps toward literacy. It is important for your child to see many different members of his family reading, so make sure both mom and dad have a chance to read to him. If he has an older sibling who can read, enlist his help.

6. Continue to expose your child to music, singing, and nursery rhymes. The rhythmic nature of music and rhymes helps your child learn to differentiate sounds and increases his cognitive function. Research suggests that learning music has a positive effect on your child's memory abilities and his ability to learn math.

7. Continue to explain the names and functions of the things your child encounters. You have many more years of answering "what?" "why?" and "how?" for your child.

8. Ask your child questions that he can answer. When reading a book, ask him to find a bird or ask him what color the turtle is. As he gets more sophisticated in his language skills, ask him what is going to happen next

in the story or ask him about his play date. Children love to share their knowledge and this helps them build language and conversation skills.

9. Never make fun of your child's incorrect pronunciation or made-up words. Your child is bound to say funny things such as *happycopter* (helicopter), *boney* (bologna), *motorbikle* (motorcycle), *ambliance* (ambulance), and *blatterfly* (butterfly)—these are just a few of the fun things we heard at our house. Enjoy his made-up words and write them down, but don't make fun of your child. This sends the message that he is doing something wrong and may cause some children to stop progressing verbally.

10. As he gets older and has more developed literacy skills, make up your own stories together. You can start a story and then ask him to add to the story. You can begin with the plot and ask him to fill in the names and characteristics of the characters in the story. Then you can add to the story. Once you have added your part, ask him to add more information. You

AHA!

The experiences gained now with talking and listening prepare your child to learn to read and write. Phonological awareness—the recognition that words are made up of separate speech sounds (CAT is made up of the sounds k a t)—is one of the most important skills for early reading. Rhyming, alliteration (big baby bouncing), and isolating sounds (F is for fish) help your child learn to segment words into separate sounds and associate the sounds with letters, which helps him to begin to learn to read and write. Finger spelling can also help your child associate the different sounds for with letters when you spell words out.

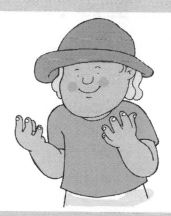

I can tell my mom that I'm wet.

might find that he takes the story in an entirely different direction.

What you are doing now is building your child's lifelong feeling for learning. If he enjoys it now, he will continue to have this experience when he enters school and will become a lifelong learner. You are teaching him knowledge, skills, dispositions, and feelings, and signing helps you do it. You are the most important teacher he will ever have.

Summary

In this chapter, we discussed:
☆ How your child is developing at two years
☆ The long-term effects of signing
☆ Continuing to sign
☆ Losing signs
☆ Encouraging speech

Bottom Line

As your child embarks on the third year of his life, enjoy the fun that comes with having a toddler who can sign and talk. Learn from him and see what he is interested in. This time in his life is short and he will never be so innocent or impressionable again. Encourage his speech and continue reading with him. Hug him and love him and watch him grow!

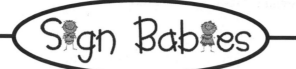
Chapter Eight

Signing with Children Who Have Special Needs

Parents whose children are not speaking on schedule often worry whether their child is delayed, because language is the primary tool that we use to understand others (receptive language) and to be understood by others (expressive language). This chapter discusses the issues specific to children with special needs and details how to adapt signing for children with special needs. Signing can be an amazing experience for children who have a speech delay, language delay, or who have more serious physical or mental limitations that make it difficult for them to express themselves.

Signing is not the answer to any condition your child might have. But it can equip you and your child with some important tools to communicate and lessen the stress you both may feel due to a lack of ability to communicate effectively. Signing will help decrease the behavior problems that occur when your child cannot effectively communicate her needs. Signing can give you both positive experiences on which to build lifelong learning habits that will improve your child's life.

In this chapter we take a look at the following:

✩ The difference between language delay and speech delay

✩ How signing can help children with special needs

✩ How to modify the baby sign language for children with special needs

IMPORTANT: Sign is used to add to your child's communication skills. Signing is *not* a substitute for talking to your child. Any time you sign, also say aloud what you are signing.

The Difference Between Language Delay and Speech Delay

As we discussed in Chapter One, *language* is how we communicate with others using words, signs, or writing and includes the types of words we use, how many words we use, how we put the words together to form thoughts, and so on. *Speech,* on the other hand, is how we pronounce words. Children can have a delay in either speech or language, or both.

Children with *mixed language delay*—a delay in understanding how language works—often have difficulty with both receptive and expressive language. For these children, using sign in addition to speech can be particularly useful for enhancing receptive language skills (understanding others). The visual cues that signs provide helps children better understand spoken language, while also providing them with vocabulary they can use.

Children with *expressive language delay* have appropriate receptive language skills appropriate for their age but are not using the appropriate number of words and are considered late talkers. Late talkers can become easily frustrated because they know and understand the same level of language as their peers, but just aren't talking yet. Signing gives these children a functional means to communicate while working toward spoken language. More than 80 percent of children who are late talkers at twenty-four months old catch up by age three with no intervention. But it can be challenging for you and your child to wait that long. Using signs can alleviate most of that frustration, because you have a communication tool that your child can use to express wants and needs.

Speech delay is most often caused by physical issues such as a lisp or stuttering, or articulation or phonological difficulties (difficulty learning associations between the visual forms of letters or pairs of letters and the sounds that they represent). Sometimes extra fluid in the ear can impair hearing and also cause speech delay, and will resolve itself once your child can hear how speech is made.

For more information on speech and language delay, see the American Speech-Language-Hearing Association (ASHA) website (www.asha.org).

AHA!

Signing adds an important visible dimension to communication. Only about 30 percent of mouthed speech is visible. If you mouth the words "I love you" without saying the words out loud, it would appear the same as if you mouthed the words "elephant shoe." By including signs in your communication, you make your communication visible as well as auditory, and help your child better understand what you are saying and be better equipped to respond and communicate with you.

Special Needs and Signing

There are several special needs conditions that cause children to have either a language delay or a speech delay, or both. The following is a description of several special needs conditions that benefit from using sign language.

Apraxia/dyspraxia/childhood apraxia of speech and developmental apraxia of speech

Apraxia is a motor coordination disorder that impacts many areas of a child's coordination—speech can be one area—and can range from mild to severe. Children with apraxia often have large vocabularies but are not understood well by others because they are inconsistent in their speech and are impacted by low tone, high tone, or physical dysfunctions. They often appear to be looking for the proper placement of their lips or tongue. They can produce words spontaneously, but when asked to repeat or label something, they can't get it to come out right because they can't coordinate the muscles in the mouth.

Research shows that when sign is used with toddlers and preschoolers who have apraxia, it takes the pressure off verbal language and relieves the frustration associated with speaking. It also makes children more willing to try to talk, which can reduce aggression associated with this frustration. For more information on this research, see www.apraxia-kids.org.

Down syndrome

Down syndrome is a genetic syndrome caused by an extra chromosome 13. Children with Down syndrome vary in their developmental progress but usually have delays in cognitive development as well as speech and language skills. Low muscle tone also contributes to delayed fine and gross motor skills as well as oral skills. Sometimes, children with Down syndrome have tongues that are enlarged, or they don't have the tactile sense to know where to place their tongues or feel where they are.

Most children with Down syndrome do not begin using verbal language until after their second birthday. This makes them perfect candidates for the use of signing. Many children with Down syndrome develop functional communication skills and do not need to rely on signing after five or six years old. Others, due to cognitive and motor delays, will rely on the use of signing throughout life to augment their verbal communication skills.

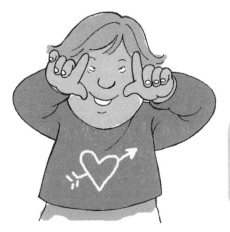

Children with Down Syndrome can sign to communicate things like **SURPRISE**.

Autism and pervasive developmental disorders

Autism is a neurological disorder characterized by delays in social interaction, language and play skills. The degree of impact for each of these delays will vary from child to child. Autism is one of five neurobiological pervasive developmental disorders (PDD) considered part of the autistic spectrum. The others are Asperger's syndrome, childhood disintegrative disorder, Rett syndrome, and PDD not otherwise specified (PDD-NOS).

Children with autism often have difficulty not just using words, but also with the social aspect of language. Signing can help these children communicate functionally with others. For a child with autism to use signing, she must be intentional in her communication—she must be trying to send you a message and must have joint attention—the ability to shift her eye gaze between you and the object you are talking about.

AHA!

You can pair signing with other communication techniques used with children with autism such as the Picture Exchange Communication System (PECS). Then you have a way to communicate when you don't have the cards you created for PECS around, because you always have your hands with you.

Cognitive delay

Children with cognitive delays tend to develop slower in many areas of development, especially thinking and play skills and speech and language skills. They will follow the same sequence of development as other children but at a slower rate. They often have shorter attention spans and are easily distracted. Behavior can become a problem in the second or third year of life because they know what they want or need, but do not have the skills to tell you yet. Signing can be used to help them with both receptive and expressive language.

Medically fragile

Children who are born premature or with extensive medical problems often show delays in their development during the first two years of life. Long hospital stays, surgical procedures, and medical equipment may interfere with a family's ability to interact with and nurture their child. These babies benefit from the use of sign because there is a greater chance they will have developmental delays in the first two years. If the medical concerns are resolved and baby maintains good health, she will probably catch up by her second birthday. Signing can help alleviate the stress of not being able to communicate during the time of delay. My son had medical issues when he was born, and we spent a lot of time at the doctor and in the hospital doing tests and so forth. He was scared that he would get poked during tests. I could let him know whether something was going to **HURT**, and he could tell me he was **SCARED** or wanted **HELP**. When the doctors saw that it calmed him down, they were astounded.

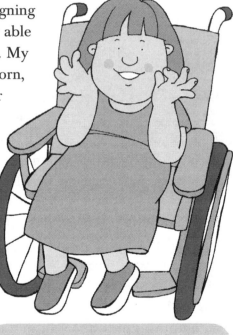

I can sign **CAT**.

Cleft palate

Children with a cleft palate are often very difficult to understand until palatal repair is complete. While the initial repair of the palate is usually done prior to the first birthday, additional surgeries may be needed to obtain intelligible speech. Signing offers children an opportunity to express themselves without the frustration of not being understood.

Tracheotomy

Children and adults with tracheotomies cannot make their voice work without a special valve in the trach tube. Many children do not have access to the valve because of ongoing respiratory issues. By using signing you can minimize delays in language by giving your child a means to communicate and develop language skills. She will then learn to talk when the trach is removed or the special valve is added to the trach tube.

Mary's daughter, Olivia, was born with cystic fibrosis and for the first one and a half years she had a trach and used signing to communicate. When Olivia was three and a half, her mom started attending sign and sing circle time classes, and Olivia had a great time learning more signing just for fun. Olivia had to have a surgery and when they were about to put her under, mom was naturally very anxious. Olivia started signing "If **YOU**'re **TIRED** and you **KNOW** it, go to **SLEEP**." This was from a song they signed and sang in circle time class ("If You're Happy and You Know It"). Olivia's mom says, "Olivia's ability to communicate with her signs at a tense time, when she couldn't use her voice, lightened the difficult situation for everyone!"

Cerebral palsy

Cerebral palsy is caused by damage to certain parts of the brain either before or during birth. Children with cerebral palsy sometimes demonstrate only mild difficulties with walking, and no other developmental areas are affected. Or they can have significant impairment in all areas of development, including cognitive and speech and language skills. If your child's motor skills are affected to the degree that she cannot move voluntarily or has difficulty moving her hands, then signing may not be possible. Look for alternate communication methods, such as a communication board. If your child has mild cerebral palsy or her arms and hands are not affected, then signing is a wonderful opportunity to expand her communication skills.

Other special needs

There are many other genetic and medical conditions that affect a child's motor skills and communication and cognitive abilities. When signing with children who have special needs, be aware of the symptoms and developmental concerns associated with the particular diagnosis. Some conditions affect cognitive and language skills while others may impact vision or hearing. Talk with your medical professionals about using signing.

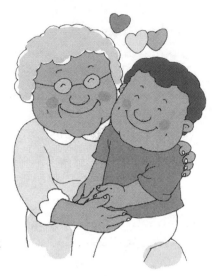

Modifying Signing for Children with Special Needs

When you are signing with a child who has special needs, you will need to adapt your strategies and your approach to meet her abilities and needs. Read *Baby Signing 1-2-3* and then keep several things in mind as you modify your signing experience.

Don't be afraid to sign

Children with special needs often require things be tweaked a bit to suit them. As you read through this book, think about how the suggestions might apply to your child. What would you need to change? Nothing about signing with babies is set in stone, so feel free to adapt it to your needs and the needs of your child. You know your child's strengths and abilities best.

If your child is severely delayed, before she can sign she must be able to bring her hands together at midline so that she can form signs, and she must understand object permanence to know something exists when it is out of sight. If your child has not reached these milestones yet, she may do so later and be able to sign in the future. Today, caregivers in adult Down syndrome programs are introducing signs to their adult patients with some success so signing does not have to occur at a specific age to have benefit for people with special needs.

Always speak when signing

You should always speak when you sign. Of course, this is also true when you sign with hearing children who are developing normally, but sometimes people forget to speak with children who have special needs. Because it might take children with special needs longer to communicate back, parents and caregivers might fall into a pattern of silence. However, the more exposure to spoken language you give to children with special needs, the better chance they have of developing the ability to speak.

Watch for approximations

All children approximate signs while they are gaining fine motor skills. However, children with special needs may always approximate their signs because their motor skills are affected by their condition. For example, children with Down syndrome may grossly approximate signs due to delays in fine motor skills or may sign in the wrong location due to gross motor difficulties. Kim Fries, a speech language pathologist and signing instructor, worked with an eighteen-month-old boy with Down syndrome who sat independently, but quite wobbly. His signs had accurate hand shapes and movements but were signed next to his leg. Because he spent so much energy trying to stay upright, he could not move his hand to his chest or face to sign without falling over.

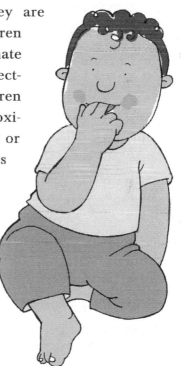

Some babies sign **EAT** by placing fingers in their mouth.

Sign specific and concrete signs

Instead of using such general signs as **MORE**, **EAT**, and **DRINK**, teach specific signs such as **MILK**, **CRACKER**, or **BANANA**. This will help you avoid a situation where your child is asking for **MORE** and you are guessing what it is that she wants. With normally developing children this is not usually a problem, but with children who have language difficulties it can be. The more specific the signs are that your child learns, the less chance of confusion and frustration. Additionally, it is better to teach signs for concrete things rather than abstract concepts, because children with special needs might not be able to make the abstract connections.

TWO CENTS

If your child's use of a sign does not help you know what she wants, needs, or is commenting on, chose an alternate sign. Teach your child as many specific signs as you can to give her a larger vocabulary to work with.

Concentrate on signs that are functional and motivating

Concentrate on functional signs that your child will be able to use immediately to get things she wants or needs. Using signs for things that your child needs will motivate her to learn to sign. Foods, favorite toys or activities and people are great signs to begin with. As discussed before, avoid general signs such as **MORE, EAT, DRINK**, or **PLAY** until your child has established a core vocabulary to avoid having to figure out what your child specifically wants.

Don't expect results overnight

Your child might take a long time to sign back, so all guesses on a timeline for communication are off. There is no way to estimate how long it might take. However, it is worth the wait and the effort to have your child be able to communicate. Before she can sign, she will probably respond to you in other ways, so look for other signs of recognition such as grunts, eye movements, changes in demeanor, or even changes in posture.

Michelle teaches children with severe disabilities in ages ranging from three to five years. One child with severe autism shakes and has ticks, but has learned to sign a few signs at home and at school (she has taught the entire class **HELP**, **SHARE**, **SORRY**, **PLEASE**, **MORE**, **EAT**, **DRINK**, **WATER**, and the signs for colors.) She says that after working with this boy for a very long time, she could see "the light go on in his eyes. He learned the sign **FRIEND** and he really got it. When I can get his attention and sign to him, he is able to focus on me—his ticks subside—and he is able to communicate. It is hard to get through to him, but it is worth it when you see the light go on—it is a heavenly thing!"

Look for help

If you have not already done so, seek help from your local resources. Work with a speech language pathologist (SLP) or an occupational therapist (OT), who understands how much signing can help children with special needs. It is a growing trend that both SLPs and OTs use signing in their therapy. Ask at the schools your child will attend whether they encourage signing. More and more schools are helping children by using signing in the classroom. If your school does not use signing now, ask them whether they would be open to having your child use sign with the teacher. You could spend some extra time with the teacher helping her to see the benefits of signing. If you need research to back up your requests, check Appendix C for a list of articles and other resources.

Keep it fun!

Make sure you don't get stressed out and don't push your child. Keep it fun and you will both have a better experience. As with most things you want to teach your special needs child, keeping the stress down and the situation fun will yield better results than pressuring your child to sign back. Use games and songs and other motivations to teach them the signs.

A Final Note on Signing with Children Who Have Special Needs

You have been blessed with a special child. Even though it takes more effort to sign with your child, the results will be worth the effort. As Jason found out, signing may sometimes be the only effective way of communicating and helping your child. "After my son Austin was diagnosed with autism at three, we got him into a special school where teachers used signing to reinforce verbal cues. Austin is now five and in a special kindergarten class where they don't seem to use the signing as much and we have kind of slacked. About six months ago, he was having a meltdown. After repeatedly telling him that we were all done and to stop, something in the back of my mind told me to get his attention. So I said and signed **STOP**, **LOOK**, **LISTEN**, **SIT**, and **ALL DONE**. The meltdown ended immediately. He wiped his face and gave me a hug and very calmly with two signs told me **MORE JUICE**. It clicked with him that we can communicate.

Ever since that day, I have worked with him and continue to learn new signs as needed to communicate with him. If a meltdown starts, 95 percent of the time it can be solved in some manner through signing and verbal communication together. The other 5 percent of the time, I understand the need and just don't give in. Signing has been nothing but a blessing for my autistic son—a blessing that opened a door into his world and allows for him to tell me what he can't put into words."

Summary

In this chapter, we discussed:

☆ The difference between language and speech delay

☆ Specific special needs and how signing can help children with these conditions

☆ How to modify the baby signing for children with special needs

Bottom Line

Signing with children who have special needs can open a door to your child's world and help open the world to your child. If your child has the physical ability to sign, it can be an amazing experience for both of you.

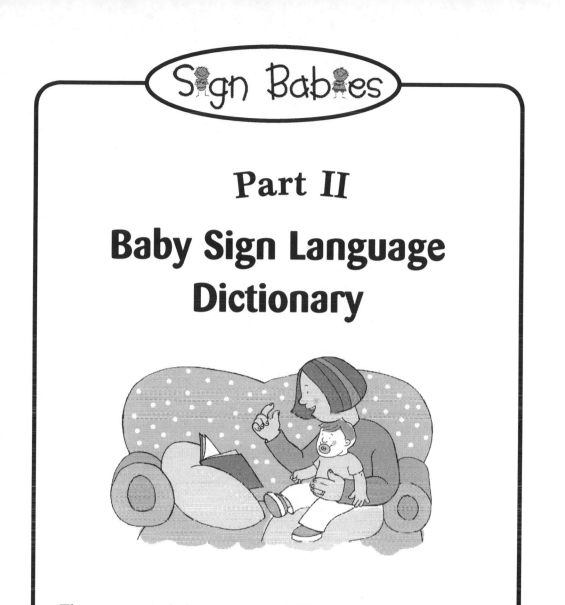

Part II

Baby Sign Language Dictionary

This section includes more than 270 signs that you can use to create two-way communication with your baby that will stop tantrums and start conversations!

The signs are organized by activity, so you can learn all the signs that are useful for a specific activity. Also, the signs to start with are shown first. Then more signs you can add are shown.

Note: If you don't find a word you want, think of a synonym or similar word for the same thing.

First Signs to Start at Four to Six Months

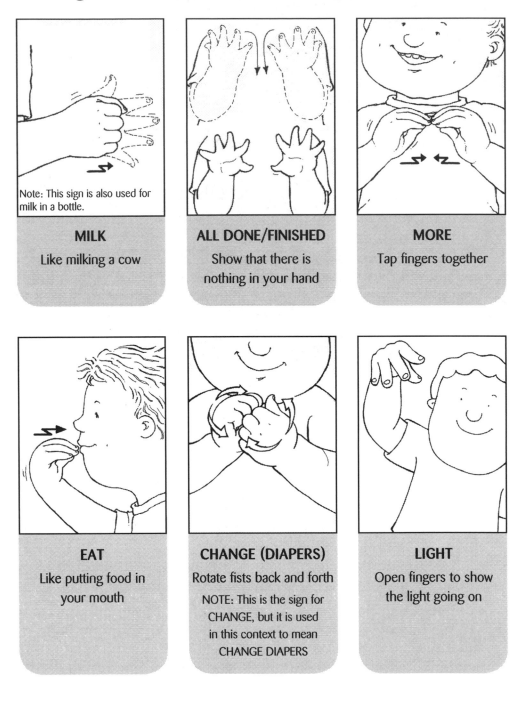

MILK

Like milking a cow

Note: This sign is also used for milk in a bottle.

ALL DONE/FINISHED

Show that there is nothing in your hand

MORE

Tap fingers together

EAT

Like putting food in your mouth

CHANGE (DIAPERS)

Rotate fists back and forth

NOTE: This is the sign for CHANGE, but it is used in this context to mean CHANGE DIAPERS

LIGHT

Open fingers to show the light going on

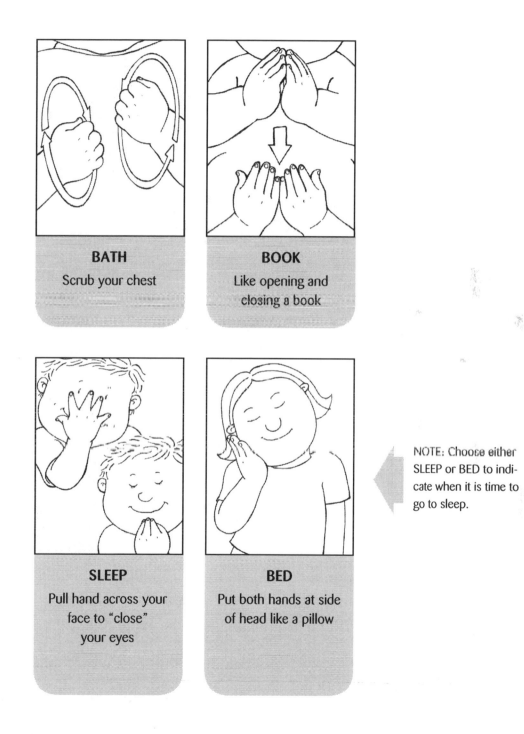

BATH
Scrub your chest

BOOK
Like opening and
closing a book

SLEEP
Pull hand across your
face to "close"
your eyes

BED
Put both hands at side
of head like a pillow

NOTE: Choose either
SLEEP or BED to indi-
cate when it is time to
go to sleep.

Diaper/Dressing Signs
Signs to start

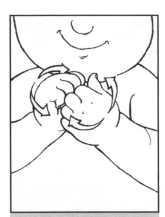

CHANGE (DIAPERS)

Rotate fists back and forth

NOTE: This is the sign for
CHANGE, but it is used
in this context to mean
CHANGE DIAPERS

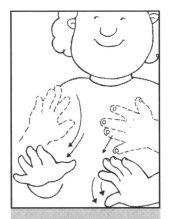

CLOTHES

Brush both hands down
your chest

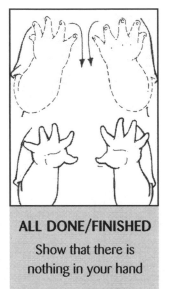

ALL DONE/FINISHED

Show that there is
nothing in your hand

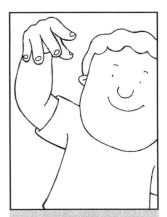

LIGHT

Open fingers to show
the light going on

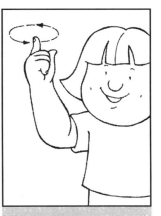

FAN

Move index finger around
in a circle above head.

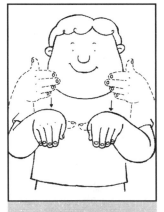

MASSAGE

Move fingers like
massaging shoulders

More signs:

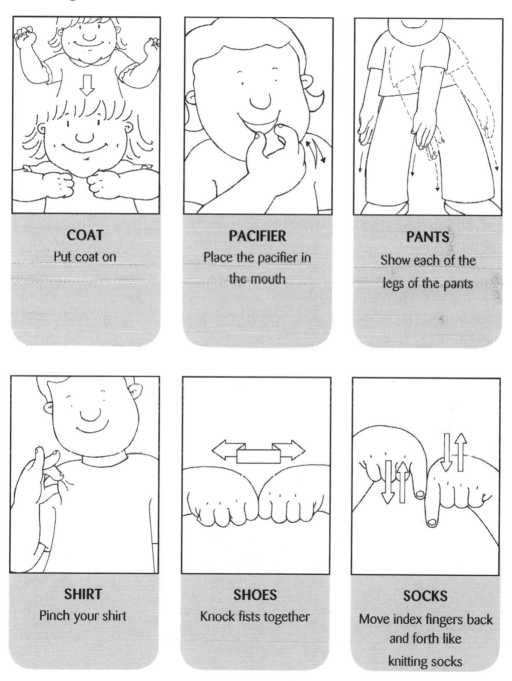

COAT
Put coat on

PACIFIER
Place the pacifier in
the mouth

PANTS
Show each of the
legs of the pants

SHIRT
Pinch your shirt

SHOES
Knock fists together

SOCKS
Move index fingers back
and forth like
knitting socks

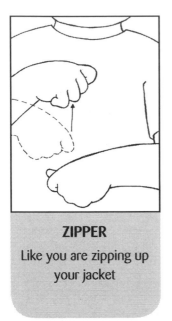

ZIPPER

Like you are zipping up
your jacket

Play and Activity Signs
Signs to start

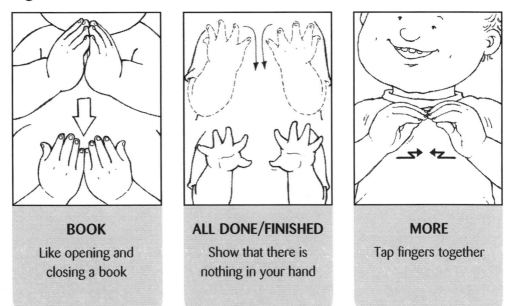

BOOK

Like opening and
closing a book

ALL DONE/FINISHED

Show that there is
nothing in your hand

MORE

Tap fingers together

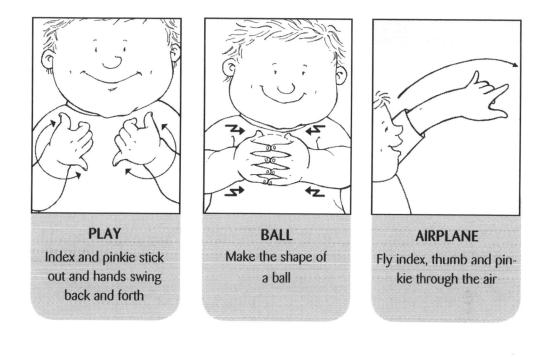

PLAY

Index and pinkie stick
out and hands swing
back and forth

BALL

Make the shape of
a ball

AIRPLANE

Fly index, thumb and pin-
kie through the air

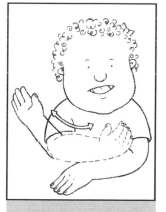

MUSIC (SING/SONG)

Like conducting music
over your arm

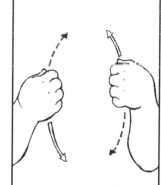

CAR

Like driving a car

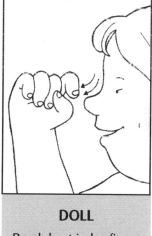

DOLL

Brush bent index finger
down nose twice

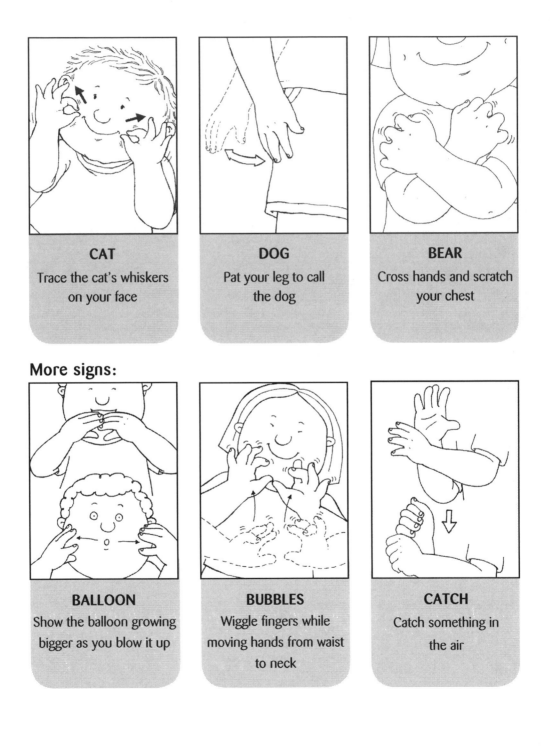

CAT
Trace the cat's whiskers
on your face

DOG
Pat your leg to call
the dog

BEAR
Cross hands and scratch
your chest

More signs:

BALLOON
Show the balloon growing
bigger as you blow it up

BUBBLES
Wiggle fingers while
moving hands from waist
to neck

CATCH
Catch something in
the air

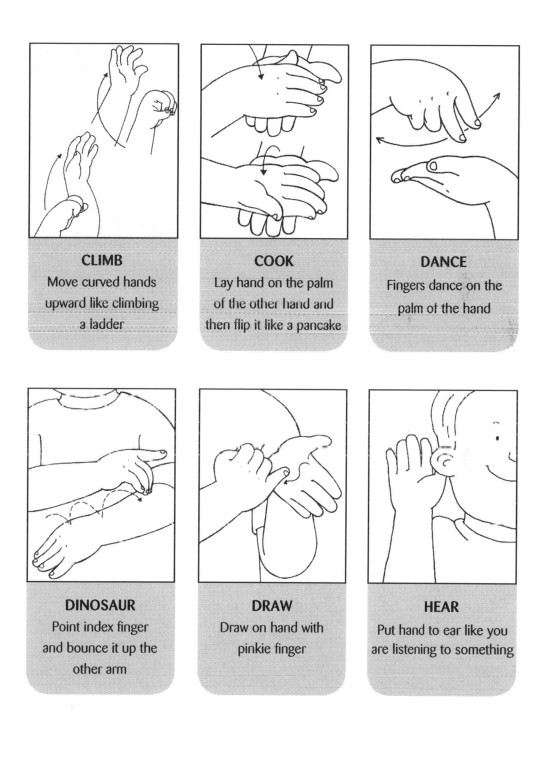

CLIMB
Move curved hands upward like climbing a ladder

COOK
Lay hand on the palm of the other hand and then flip it like a pancake

DANCE
Fingers dance on the palm of the hand

DINOSAUR
Point index finger and bounce it up the other arm

DRAW
Draw on hand with pinkie finger

HEAR
Put hand to ear like you are listening to something

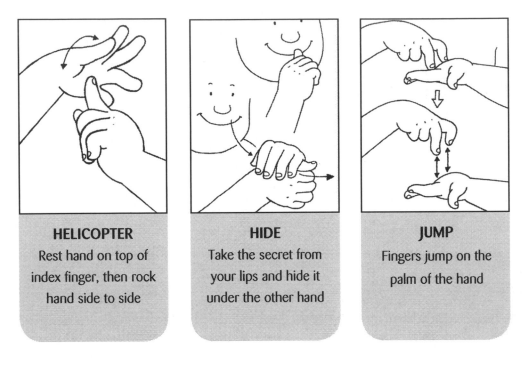

HELICOPTER
Rest hand on top of
index finger, then rock
hand side to side

HIDE
Take the secret from
your lips and hide it
under the other hand

JUMP
Fingers jump on the
palm of the hand

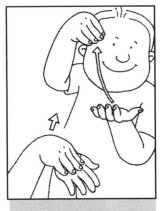

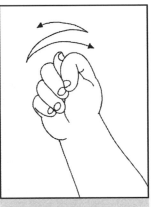

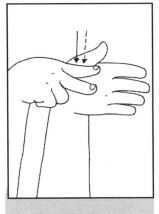

LEARN
Grab information and
put it into your head

POTTY
Tuck your thumb under
your index finger and
then shake it

READ
Index and middle
fingers move over other
hand like reading book

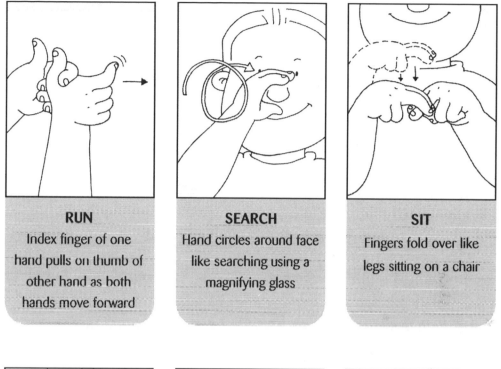

RUN

Index finger of one hand pulls on thumb of other hand as both hands move forward

SEARCH

Hand circles around face like searching using a magnifying glass

SIT

Fingers fold over like legs sitting on a chair

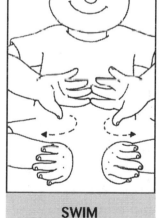

SWIM

Move hands like you are swimming

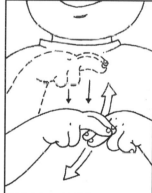

SWING

Fingers fold over like legs sitting on a chair, then swing back and forth

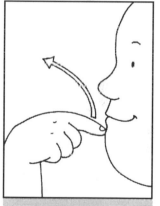

TELL

Index finger starts under chin and thrusts out

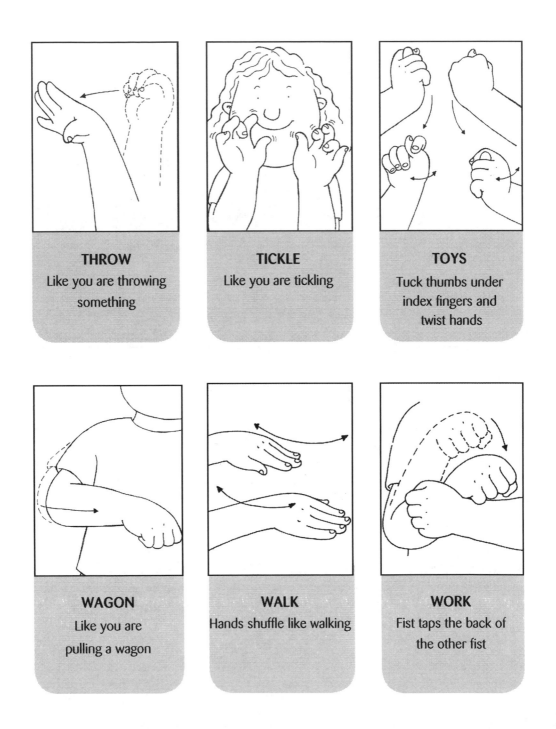

THROW
Like you are throwing
something

TICKLE
Like you are tickling

TOYS
Tuck thumbs under
index fingers and
twist hands

WAGON
Like you are
pulling a wagon

WALK
Hands shuffle like walking

WORK
Fist taps the back of
the other fist

Bath Signs/Hygiene Signs
Signs to start

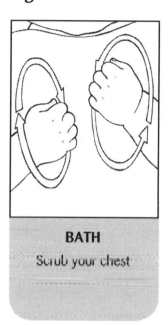

BATH

Scrub your chest

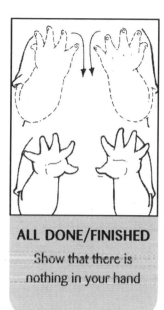

ALL DONE/FINISHED

Show that there is
nothing in your hand

More signs:

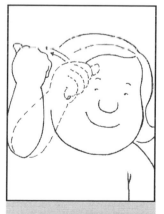

BRUSH HAIR

Like you are brushing
your hair

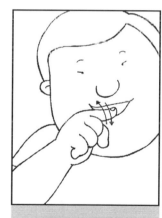

BRUSH TEETH

Like you are brushing
your teeth

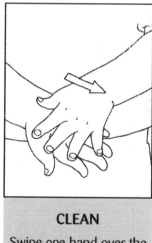

CLEAN

Swipe one hand over the
other like cleaning

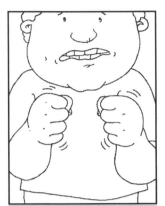

COLD
Make two fists and shake
them like you're shivering

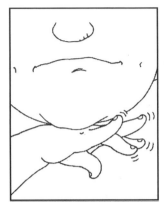

DIRTY
Wiggle fingers
under chin

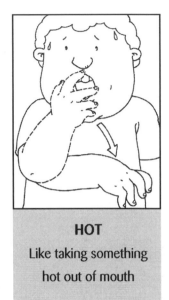

HOT
Like taking something
hot out of mouth

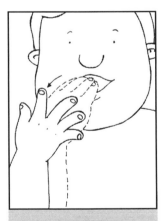

WARM
Open fingers at mouth
like warm breath
moving out of mouth

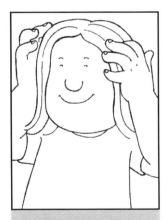

WASH HAIR
Like washing your hair

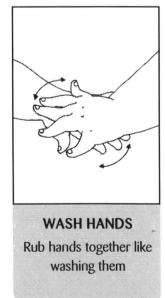

WASH HANDS
Rub hands together like
washing them

Bedtime Signs
Signs to start

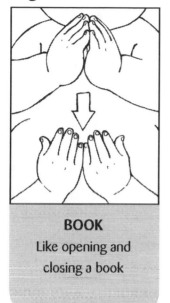

BOOK
Like opening and
closing a book

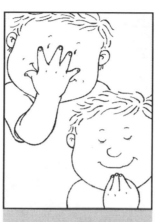

SLEEP
Pull hand across your
face to "close" your eyes

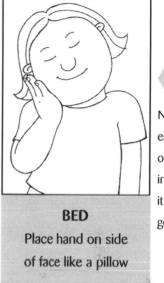

BED
Place hand on side
of face like a pillow

NOTE: Choose
either SLEEP
or BED to
indicate when
it is time to
go to sleep.

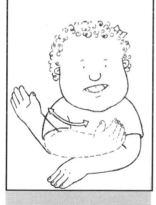

MUSIC (SING)
Like conducting music
over your arm

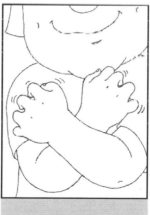

BEAR
Cross hands and scratch
your chest

More signs

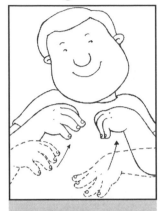

BLANKET
Move hands like pulling a blanket up to your chest

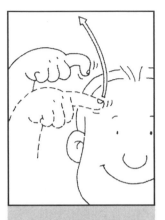

DREAM
Index finger wiggle out from head

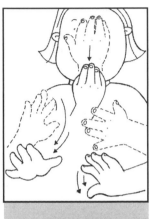

PAJAMAS
Use two signs SLEEP and CLOTHES

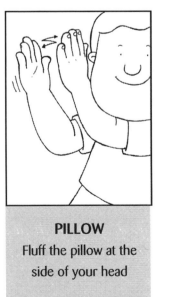

PILLOW
Fluff the pillow at the side of your head

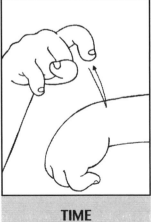

TIME
Tap "wristwatch"

Food Signs
Signs to start

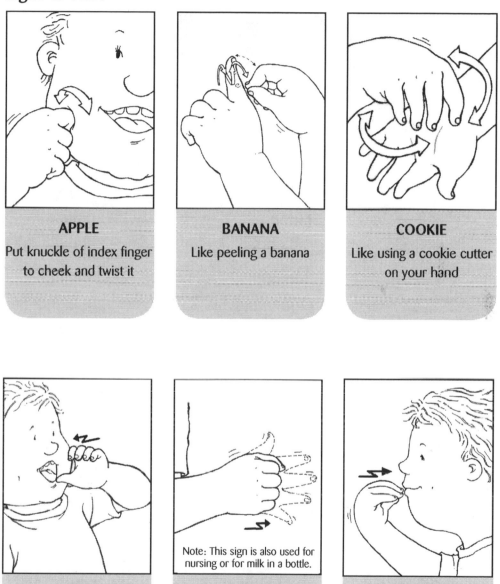

APPLE
Put knuckle of index finger
to cheek and twist it

BANANA
Like peeling a banana

COOKIE
Like using a cookie cutter
on your hand

DRINK
Like drinking from a cup

Note: This sign is also used for
nursing or for milk in a bottle.

MILK
Like milking a cow

EAT
Like putting food
in your mouth

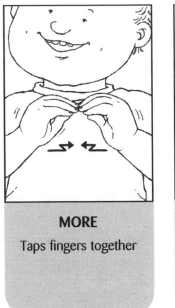

MORE

Taps fingers together

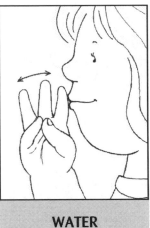

WATER

Tap three middle
fingers at your lips

More signs

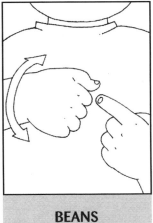

BEANS

Twist the bean open

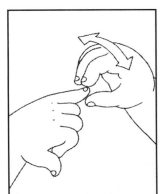

BERRY

Twist the berry off
your pinkie finger

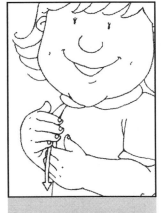

BREAD

Like slicing a loaf
of bread

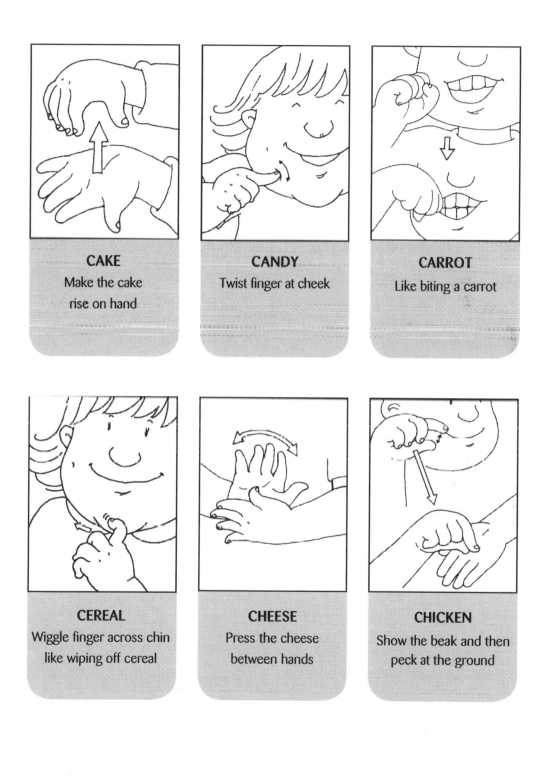

CAKE
Make the cake
rise on hand

CANDY
Twist finger at cheek

CARROT
Like biting a carrot

CEREAL
Wiggle finger across chin
like wiping off cereal

CHEESE
Press the cheese
between hands

CHICKEN
Show the beak and then
peck at the ground

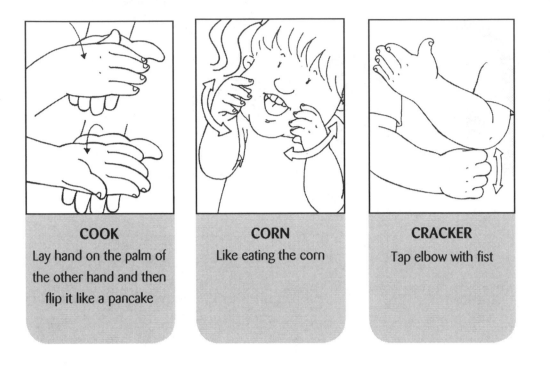

COOK
Lay hand on the palm of
the other hand and then
flip it like a pancake

CORN
Like eating the corn

CRACKER
Tap elbow with fist

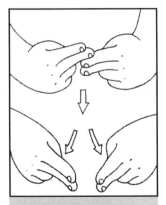

EGG
Tap fingers togheter
ike breaking and
opening an egg

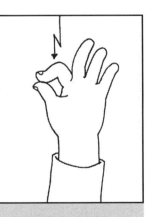

FRENCH FRIES
Bounce index finger and
thumb in the air

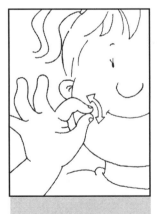

FRUIT
Twist thumb and index
finger at the side of the
mouth

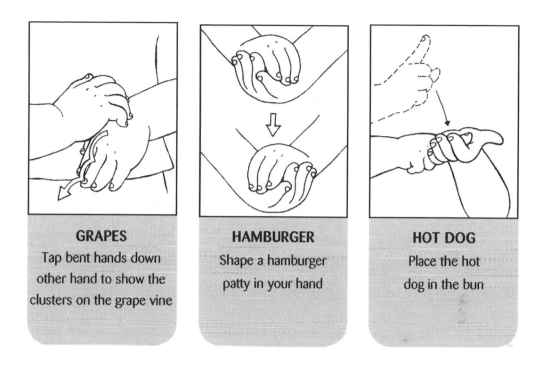

GRAPES
Tap bent hands down
other hand to show the
clusters on the grape vine

HAMBURGER
Shape a hamburger
patty in your hand

HOT DOG
Place the hot
dog in the bun

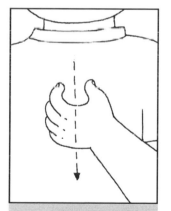

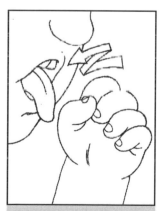

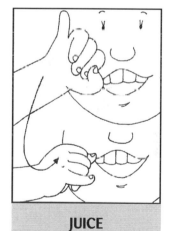

HUNGRY
Move curved hand down
chest to show food
moving down to stomach

ICE CREAM
Move "ice cream cone" in
front of mouth to lick it

JUICE
Trace the letter
"J" with pinkie

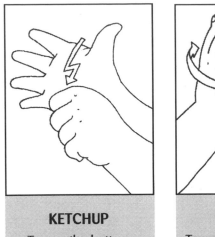

KETCHUP

Tap on the bottom
of the bottle

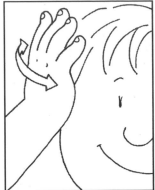

LETTUCE

Tap palm at the head to
show a "head" of lettuce

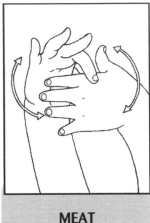

MEAT

Pinch skin between
thumb and index finger
and wiggle pinching hand

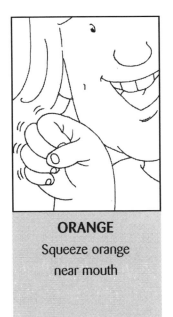

ORANGE

Squeeze orange
near mouth

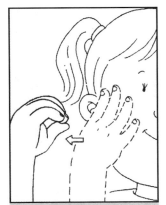

PEACH

Feel the peac fuzz
on your cheek

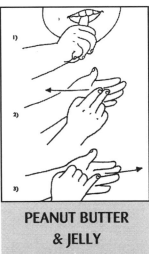

**PEANUT BUTTER
& JELLY**

(1) Brush thumb against
teeth, (2) Butter bread
with two fingers, (3)
Spread jelly with pinkie

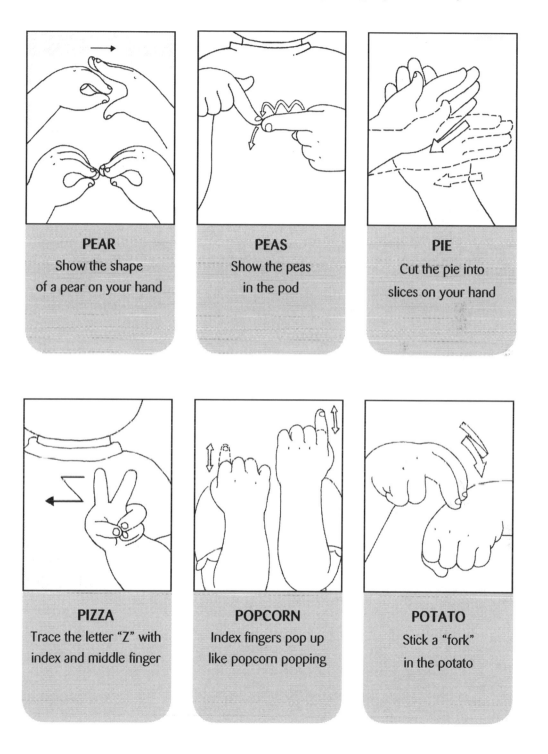

PEAR
Show the shape
of a pear on your hand

PEAS
Show the peas
in the pod

PIE
Cut the pie into
slices on your hand

PIZZA
Trace the letter "Z" with
index and middle finger

POPCORN
Index fingers pop up
like popcorn popping

POTATO
Stick a "fork"
in the potato

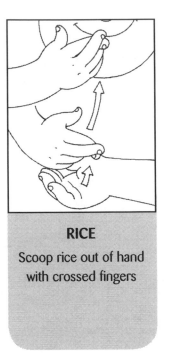

RICE

Scoop rice out of hand
with crossed fingers

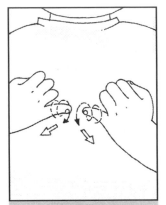

SPAGHETTI

Circle pinkies as they
move away from
each other

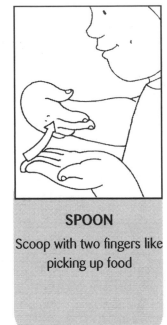

SPOON

Scoop with two fingers like
picking up food

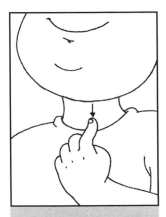

THIRSTY

Run index finger
down throat

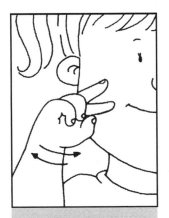

VEGETABLE

Twist index and
middle finger at
the side of the mouth

Animal Signs
Signs to start

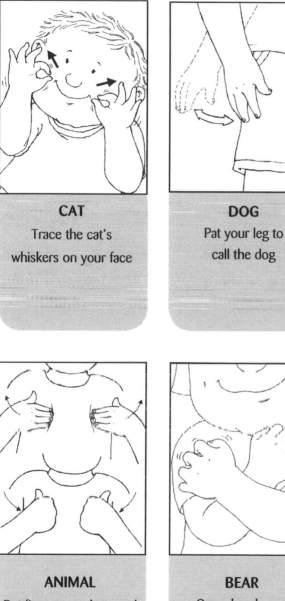

CAT
Trace the cat's
whiskers on your face

DOG
Pat your leg to
call the dog

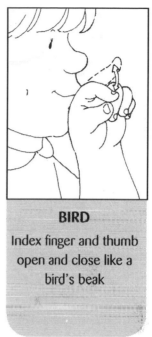

BIRD
Index finger and thumb
open and close like a
bird's beak

ANIMAL
Put fingers on chest and
move hands like wings

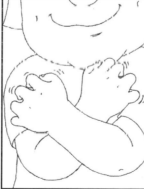

BEAR
Cross hands and
scratch your chest

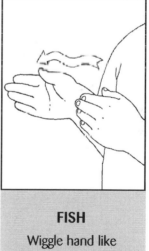

FISH
Wiggle hand like
a fish swimming

More signs

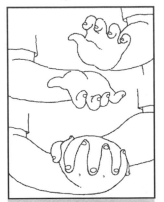

ALLIGATOR

Open and close two
hands together like
alligator's mouth

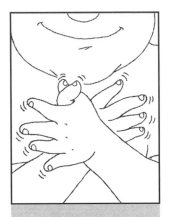

BUTTERFLY

Hook thumbs together and
flap hands like wings

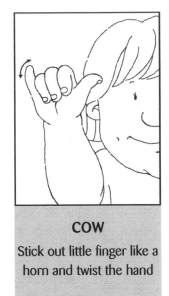

COW

Stick out little finger like a
horn and twist the hand

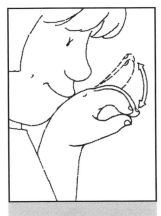

DUCK

Index and middle
finger tap thumb like
a duck's bill

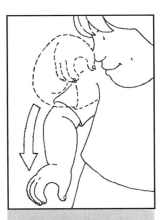

ELEPHANT

Move curved hand
from nose down to
show elephant's trunk

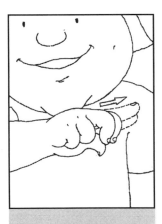

FROG

Flick fingers under chin
like frog's throat puffing

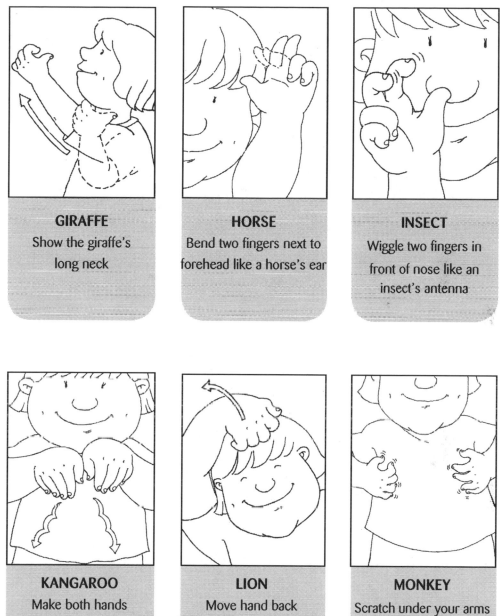

GIRAFFE
Show the giraffe's long neck

HORSE
Bend two fingers next to forehead like a horse's ear

INSECT
Wiggle two fingers in front of nose like an insect's antenna

KANGAROO
Make both hands hop like a kangaroo

LION
Move hand back over the head to show the lion's mane

MONKEY
Scratch under your arms like a monkey

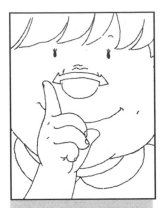

MOUSE

Rub index finger
across scrunched nose

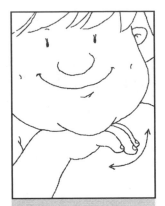

PIG

Open and close
hand under chin

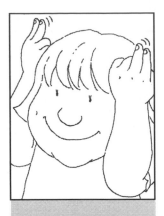

RABBIT

Wiggle fingers
like rabbit ears

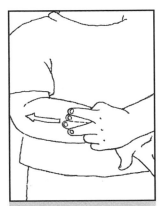

SHEEP

Use a scissors motion
to "shear wool"
on inside of arm

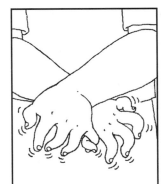

SPIDER

Interlock pinkies
and wiggle fingers

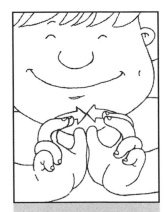

SQUIRREL

Tap two fingers like
squirrel's teeth
opening and closing

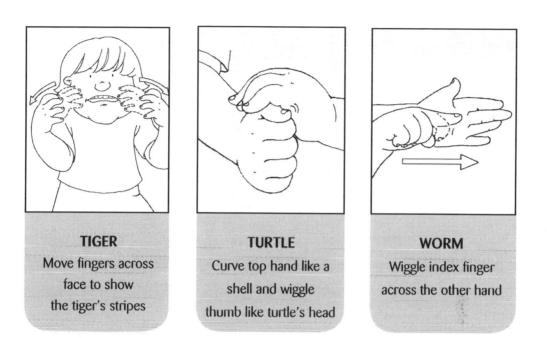

TIGER
Move fingers across
face to show
the tiger's stripes

TURTLE
Curve top hand like a
shell and wiggle
thumb like turtle's head

WORM
Wiggle index finger
across the other hand

Family and Friend Signs
Signs to start

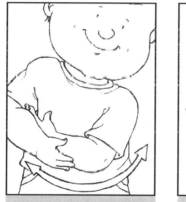

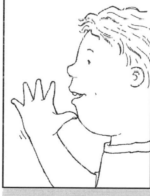

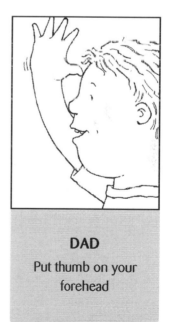

BABY
Like rocking a baby

MOM
Put thumb on your chin

DAD
Put thumb on your
forehead

More signs

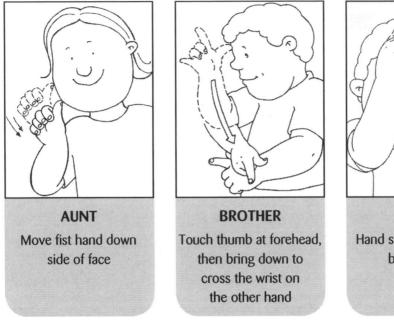

AUNT

Move fist hand down side of face

BROTHER

Touch thumb at forehead, then bring down to cross the wrist on the other hand

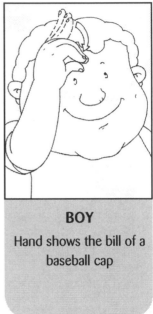

BOY

Hand shows the bill of a baseball cap

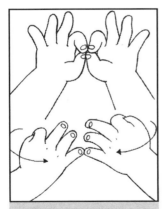

FAMILY

Thumb and fingers touch, then move to make a family circle

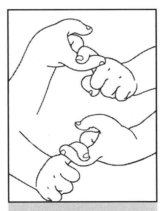

FRIEND

Hook index fingers to gether and then switch them

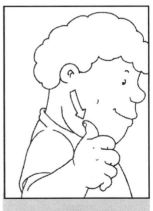

GIRL

Thumb traces the girl's bonnet strings

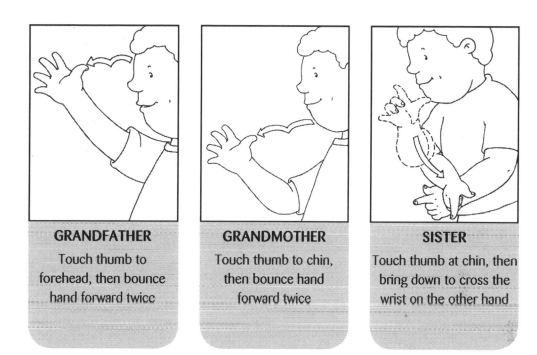

GRANDFATHER

Touch thumb to forehead, then bounce hand forward twice

GRANDMOTHER

Touch thumb to chin, then bounce hand forward twice

SISTER

Touch thumb at chin, then bring down to cross the wrist on the other hand

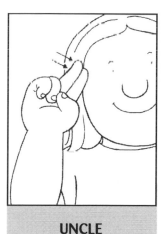

UNCLE

Move index and middle finger up and down at the temple

Emotions Signs
Signs to start

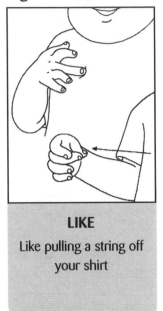

LIKE

Like pulling a string off your shirt

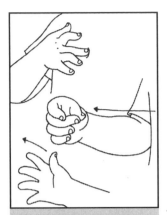

DON'T LIKE

Pull string off shirt and throw away

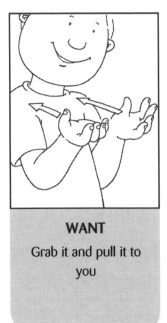

WANT

Grab it and pull it to you

More signs

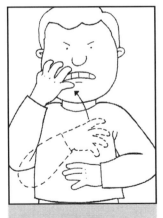

ANGRY

Move claw-like hand from angry face to chest

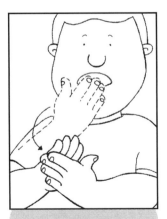

BAD

Move hand from face to slap the other hand

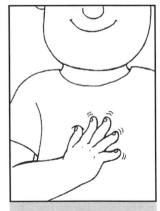

COOL

Put thumb on chest and wiggle fingers

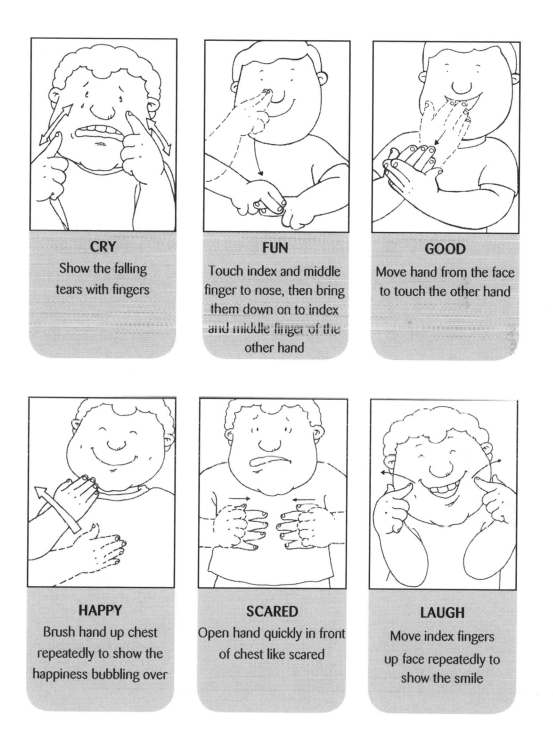

CRY
Show the falling
tears with fingers

FUN
Touch index and middle
finger to nose, then bring
them down on to index
and middle finger of the
other hand

GOOD
Move hand from the face
to touch the other hand

HAPPY
Brush hand up chest
repeatedly to show the
happiness bubbling over

SCARED
Open hand quickly in front
of chest like scared

LAUGH
Move index fingers
up face repeatedly to
show the smile

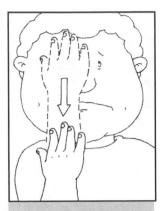

SAD

Move hand over
your sad face in a
downward direction

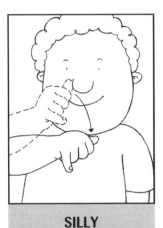

SILLY

Extend thumb and pinkie,
then rub thumb across
nose a few times

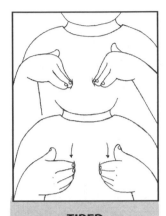

TIRED

Rest fingertips at
shoulders, then let
them fall forward to
show you are tired

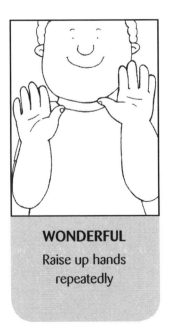

WONDERFUL

Raise up hands
repeatedly

Manner Signs
Signs to start

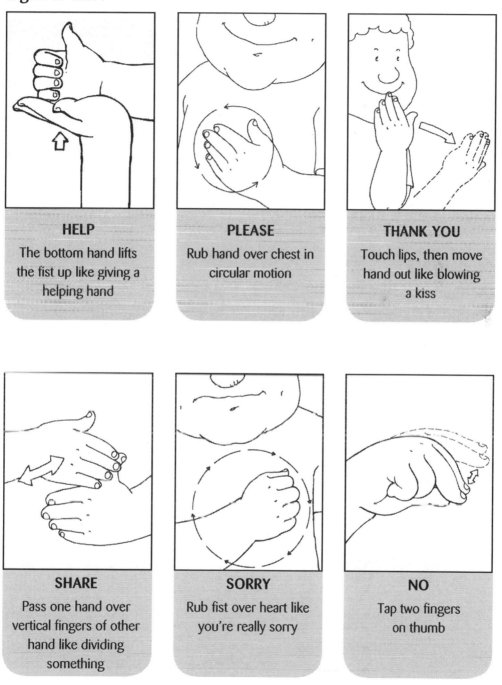

HELP

The bottom hand lifts the fist up like giving a helping hand

PLEASE

Rub hand over chest in circular motion

THANK YOU

Touch lips, then move hand out like blowing a kiss

SHARE

Pass one hand over vertical fingers of other hand like dividing something

SORRY

Rub fist over heart like you're really sorry

NO

Tap two fingers on thumb

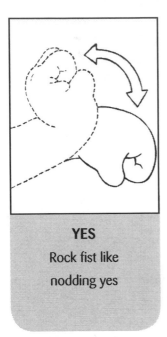

YES

Rock fist like
nodding yes

More signs

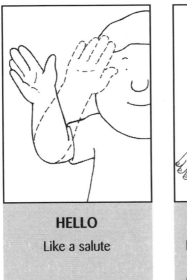

HELLO

Like a salute

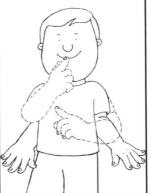

QUIET

Put finger to lips to say
"Quiet", then move
hands out to show that
everything gets quiet

NOTE: You can sign
just the finger at the
lips too, but some
moms have found that
including the hands
moving out helps their
children to calm down.

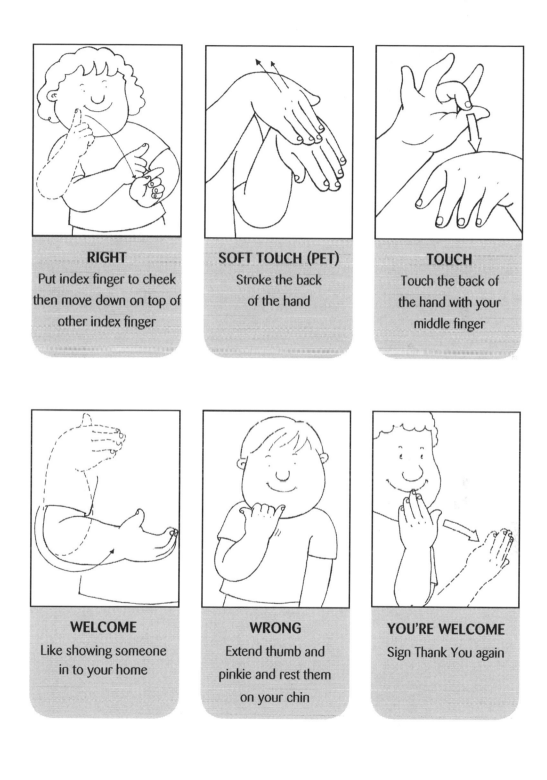

RIGHT
Put index finger to cheek
then move down on top of
other index finger

SOFT TOUCH (PET)
Stroke the back
of the hand

TOUCH
Touch the back of
the hand with your
middle finger

WELCOME
Like showing someone
in to your home

WRONG
Extend thumb and
pinkie and rest them
on your chin

YOU'RE WELCOME
Sign Thank You again

Health and Safety Signs
Signs to start

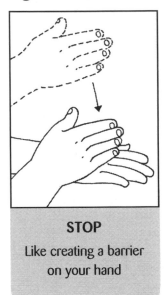

STOP

Like creating a barrier
on your hand

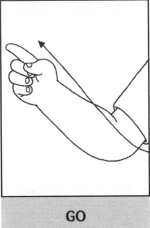

GO

Index finger point the
way you want to go

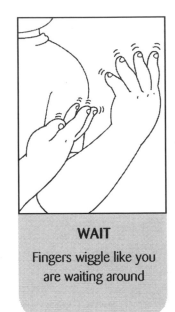

WAIT

Fingers wiggle like you
are waiting around

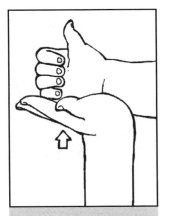

HELP

The bottom hand lifts
the fist up like giving a
helping hand

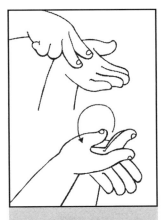

FALL DOWN

Index and middle fingers
stand on the hand and
then "fall down"

More signs

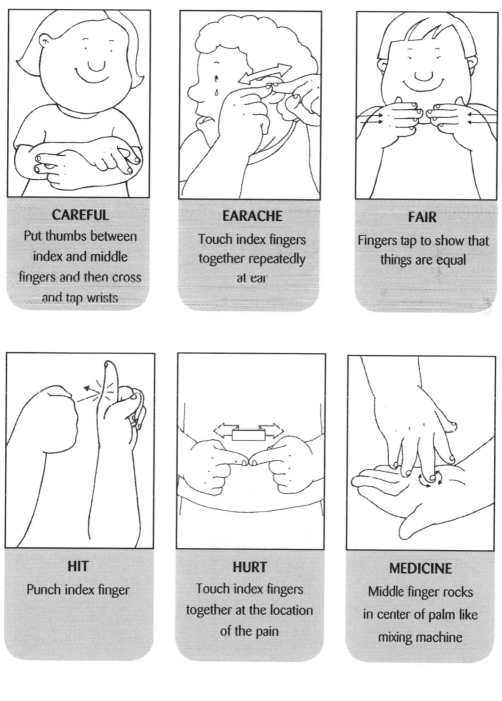

CAREFUL
Put thumbs between index and middle fingers and then cross and tap wrists

EARACHE
Touch index fingers together repeatedly at ear

FAIR
Fingers tap to show that things are equal

HIT
Punch index finger

HURT
Touch index fingers together at the location of the pain

MEDICINE
Middle finger rocks in center of palm like mixing machine

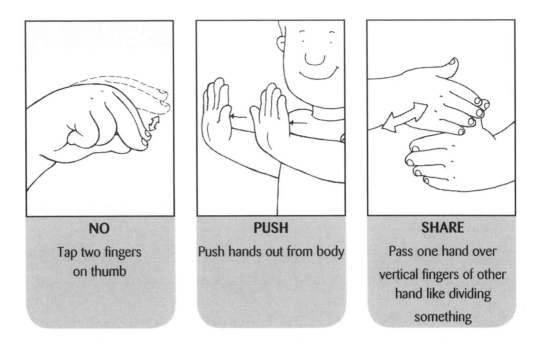

NO
Tap two fingers
on thumb

PUSH
Push hands out from body

SHARE
Pass one hand over
vertical fingers of other
hand like dividing
something

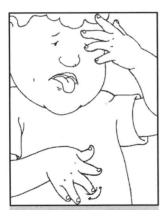

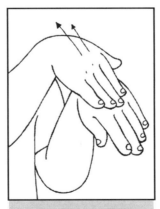

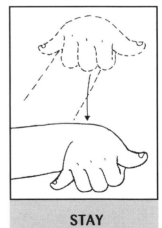

SICK
Touch middle finger
to forehead and
stomach and twist

SOFT TOUCH (PET)
Stroke the back
of the hand

STAY
Thumb and pinkie stick
out as hand moves
down firmly

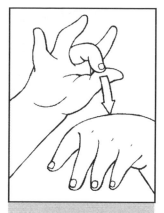

TOUCH
Touch the back of
the hand with your
middle finger

Household Signs
Signs to start

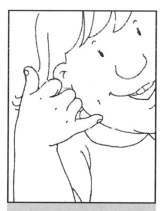

TELEPHONE
Index and pinkie make a
phone at the ear

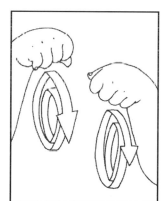

BIKE
Like pedaling a bike

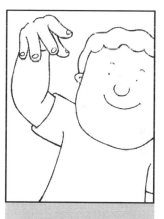

LIGHT ON
Open fingers to show
the light going on

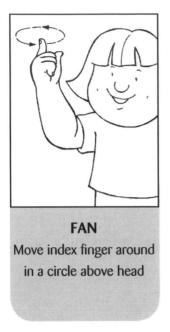

FAN
Move index finger around
in a circle above head

More signs

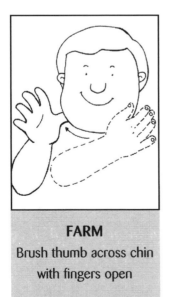

FARM
Brush thumb across chin
with fingers open

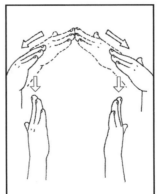

HOUSE
Make a house shape
with your hands

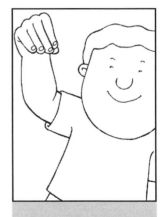

LIGHTS OFF
Close fingers to show
the light going off

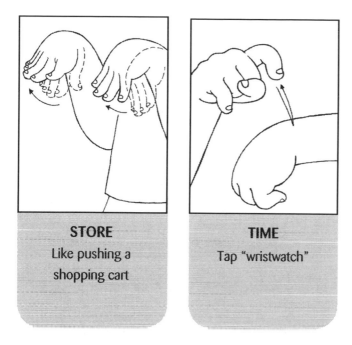

STORE
Like pushing a
shopping cart

TIME
Tap "wristwatch"

Weather/Outdoor Signs
Signs to Start

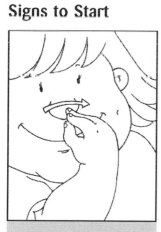

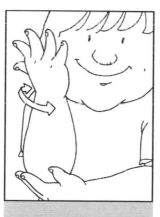

FLOWER
Smell the flower
at your nose

TREE
Arm and hand form a
tree, then hand twists
like swaying in the wind

More signs

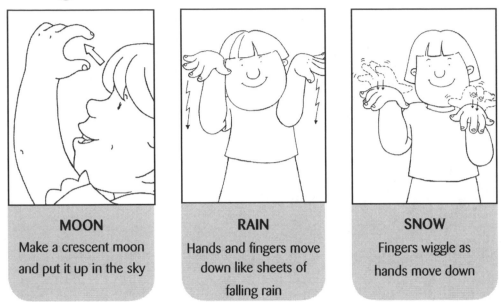

MOON
Make a crescent moon
and put it up in the sky

RAIN
Hands and fingers move
down like sheets of
falling rain

SNOW
Fingers wiggle as
hands move down

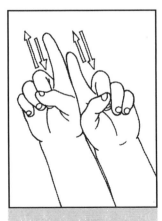

STARS
Move index fingers
back and forth like
shooting stars

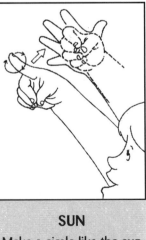

SUN
Make a circle like the sun
and then show its rays

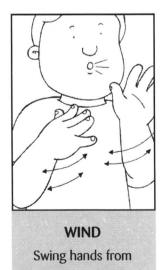

WIND
Swing hands from
side to side

Descriptor Signs
Signs to start

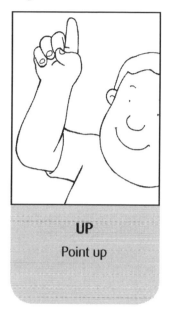

UP

Point up

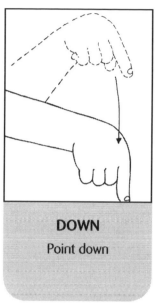

DOWN

Point down

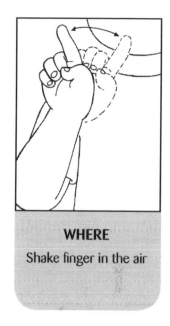

WHERE

Shake finger in the air

More signs

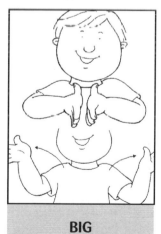

BIG

Open hands to show how
big you want to describe

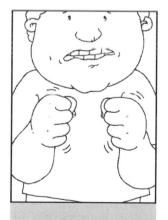

COLD

Make two fists and shake
them like you're shivering

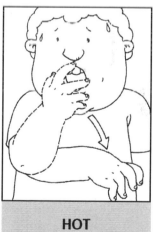

HOT

Like taking something
hot out of mouth

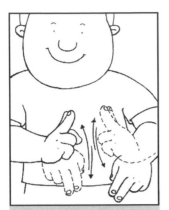

HURRY

Index and middle
fingers move up
and down quickly

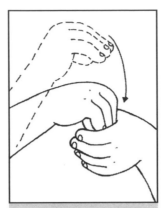

IN/INSIDE

Like putting something
in a container

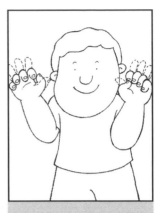

A LOT

Open and close hands
repeatedly to show that
there is a lot

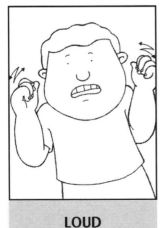

LOUD

Shake fists at side of head

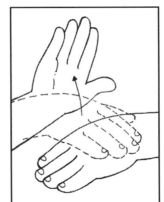

OFF

Lift hand off the back
of the other hand

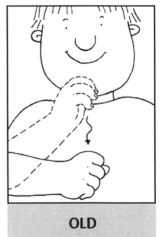

OLD

Show a man's wavy
beard

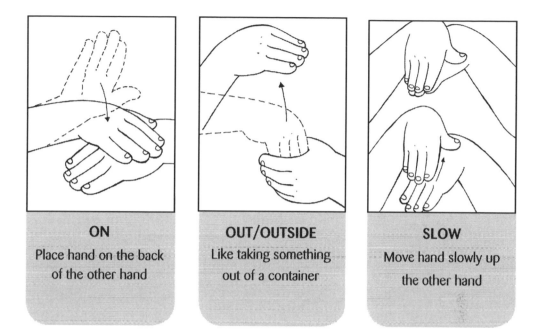

ON
Place hand on the back
of the other hand

OUT/OUTSIDE
Like taking something
out of a container

SLOW
Move hand slowly up
the other hand

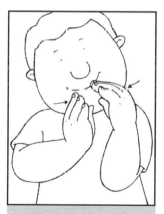

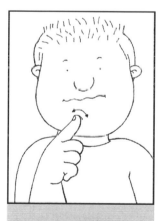

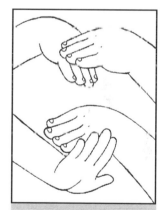

SMALL
Move hands close
together to show how
small you want to
describe

SOUR
Make a sour face and
twist index finger under
chin

UNDER
Slide hand under
the other hand

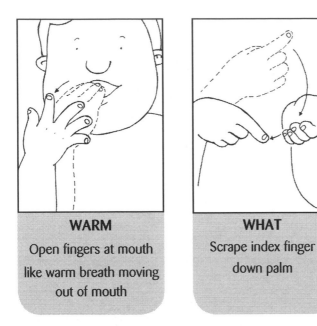

WARM

Open fingers at mouth like warm breath moving out of mouth

WHAT

Scrape index finger down palm

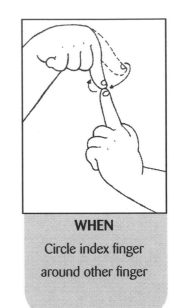

WHEN

Circle index finger around other finger

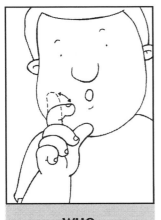

WHO

Make "O" with lips, then put thumb at chin and bend index finger repeatedly

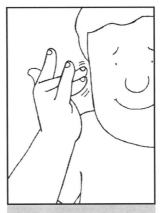

WHY

Tap middle fingers to head

Alphabet Signs

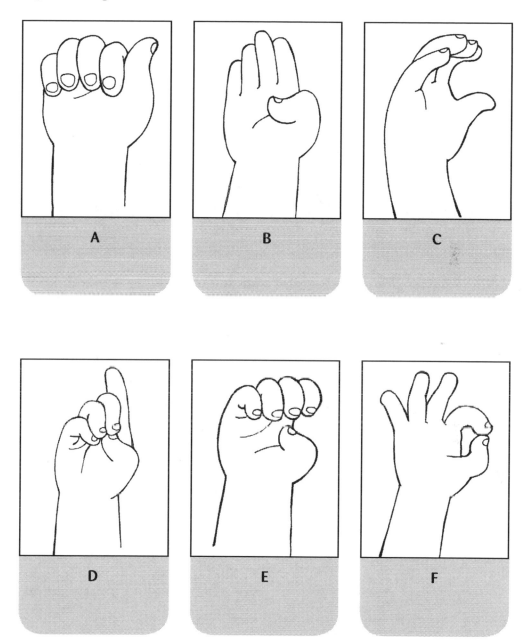

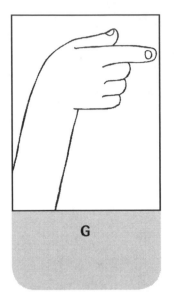

G

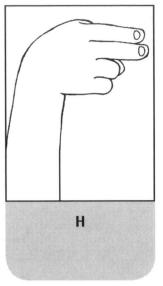

H

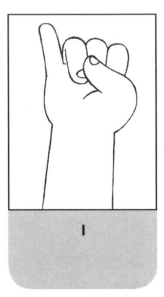

I

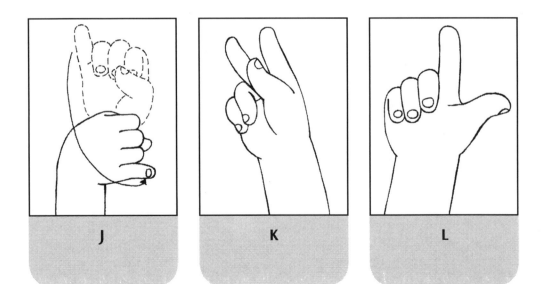

J

K

L

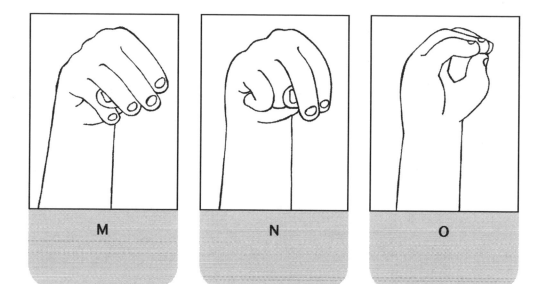

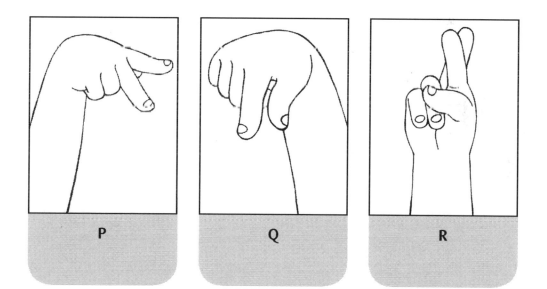

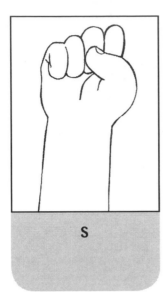

S

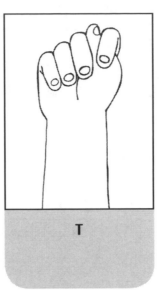

T

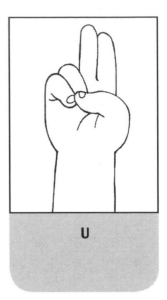

U

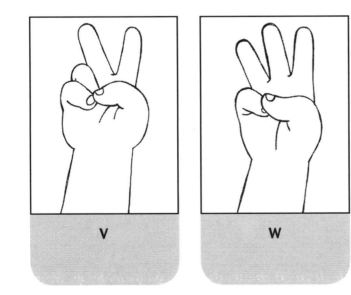

V

W

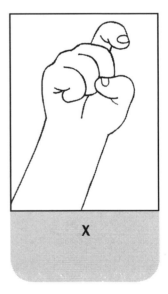

X

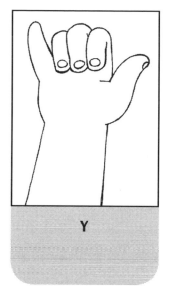

Y

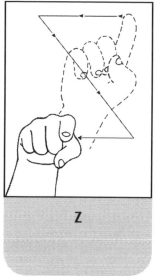

Z

Number Signs

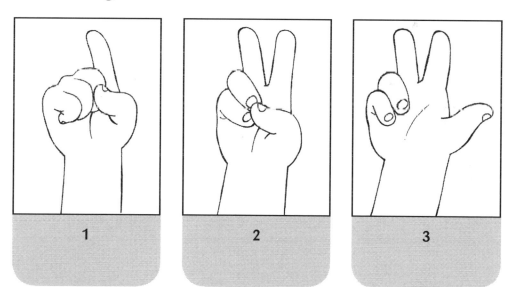

1

2

3

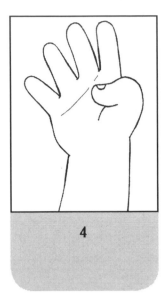

4

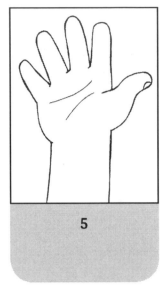

5

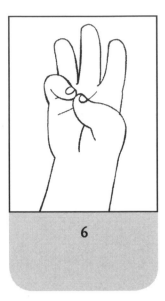

6

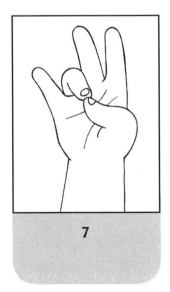

7

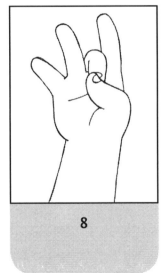

8

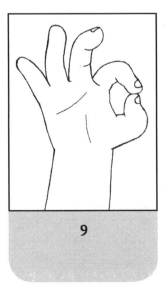

9

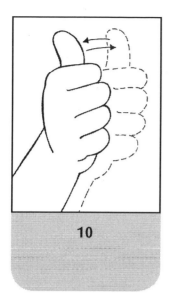

10

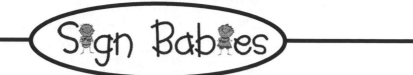

Appendix A

Quick Review of Developmental Stages by Age

Age	Motor	Language
0–3	• lifts head and chest when lying on stomach • grasps rattle or finger • wiggles and kicks with arms and legs • rolls over (stomach to back) • sits with support	• responds to mother's high-pitched voice • cries (with tears) to communicate pain, fear, discomfort, or loneliness • babbles or coos
4–7	• reaches for objects • uses finger and thumb to pick up an object • develops a rhythm for feeding, eliminating, sleeping, and being awake • rolls from back to stomach and stomach to back • transfers objects from one hand to the other	• distinguishes sounds • cries in different ways to say she is hurt, wet, hungry, or lonely • makes noises to voice displeasure or satisfaction • babbles expressively as if talking • imitates sounds, actions, and facial expressions made by others • squeals, laughs, babbles, smiles in response • may make first sign
8–12	• mastered the pincer grasp • continues to explore • continues to explore everything by mouth • crawls well • pulls self to a standing position • stands alone and walks holding onto furniture for support	• makes first sign • says first word • says da-da and ma-ma or equivalent

Cognitive	Social	Signing
• explores objects with mouth • plays with fingers, hands, toes • reacts to sound of voice, rattle, bell • turns head toward bright colors and lights • recognizes bottle or breast	• loves to be touched and held close • returns a smile • responds to peek-a-boo games • responds to a shaking rattle or bell	*You can sign with your baby at this time, but she cannot sign back yet. She may recognize and respond to your signs. If you feel tired or stressed, focus on bonding with your baby instead of signing.*
• recognizes and looks for familiar voices and sounds • learns by using senses like smell, taste, touch, sight, hearing • looks for ball rolled out of sight • searches for toys hidden under a blanket, basket, or container • explores objects by touching, shaking, banging, and mouthing • enjoys dropping objects over edge of chair or crib	• responds to own name • spends a great deal of time watching and observing • responds differently to strangers and family members • likes to be tickled and touched • smiles at own reflection in mirror • raises arms as a sign to be held • recognizes family member names • responds to distress of others by showing distress or crying • shows mild to severe anxiety at separation from parent	• responds to signs with verbal and physical cues • may make one or two signs like MORE, MILK, or EAT • understands as many as fifteen distinct signs
• "dances" or bounces to music • interested in picture books • pays attention to conversations • claps hands, waves bye, if prompted • likes to place objects inside one another	• responds to name • likes to watch self in mirror • expresses separation anxiety • pushes away something she does not want	• makes first sign back • masters several signs • may sign two-sign combinations • wants to know the signs for everything he sees

Age	Motor	Language
13–18	• stands and walks alone • jumps and dances • increases manual dexterity	• responds to simple commands • understands at least ten to fifteen regularly used words; more if she is signing • speaks one or more words • identifies objects correctly
19–24	• uses hands more to develop fine motor skills • likes to draw • likes to use a spoon or fork	• speaks several words • may have experienced a language explosion and speak more than fifty words • responds to more complex commands • understands about 200 words
25+	• dresses and feeds herself • strings beads, uses paint brushes, cuts with scissors, draws with crayons • throws and kicks a ball, hops on one foot, pedals a tricycle, and climbs up and down a small slide	• understands 400 words at thirty months and up to 800 words at thirty-six months • speaks in three- to five-word sentences • uses past tense correctly most of the time

Cognitive	Social	Signing
• recalls things that occurred a few hours or days ago • enjoys repetition as a tool for learning	• imitates adult actions such as drinking from a cup, talking on phone • has a wider range of emotions • has a hard time controlling her emotions	• signs several signs • uses signs to explain what she sees as well as what she needs • may sign and speak to communicate a thought
• learns through experience more than stories • understands that symbols stand for objects • understands symbolic thought and pretend play	• imitates adult actions such as drinking from a cup, talking on phone • can play alone for longer periods of time • may become possessive of toys • may be able to learn the beginning of sharing	• signs and speaks at the same time • gradually drops signs for the words she can speak clearly
• asks Why frequently • asks questions when you read books • may recognize letters and some simplewords	• plays by herself • plays imaginative games and thinks of new ways to use toys • can share toys • learning to control very strong emotions • pushes boundaries to understand the rules	• signs and speaks at the same time • gradually drops signs for the words she can speak clearly • may keep a few signs she especially loves

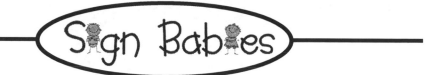

Appendix B

How Signing with Babies Started

Sign language is not new. There have been records of sign languages back to the ancient Babylonians. People have even recognized the effect that signing had on hearing siblings or hearing children in deaf families. As far back as the 1800s, researchers reported that the hearing siblings of deaf families could sign and could even read better than their hearing counterparts who did not grow up signing.

The real signing with babies movement started in the 1980s. Joseph Garcia, who was not raised within Deaf culture, had become friends with many deaf people and had even become an interpreter. During his time with deaf families, he had noticed that even the hearing children of deaf adults could sign at an early age and had an easy time communicating what they needed. He decided to research the communication abilities of hearing babies whose parents taught them basic American Sign Language (ASL) signs to communicate. He was encouraged to publish his findings, but it was not until the 1990s that his book *SIGN with your BABY* was published and helped teach thousands of parents how to sign with their hearing babies.

This is actually the book that helped me start signing with my son. I am very grateful to Dr. Garcia for his book and for his love of people and, especially children. I have had the chance to meet him, and he is one of the most engaging and loving people I have ever been with. He has helped thousands of families to have better relationships with their children.

In the 1980s, two women at the University of California, Davis, Linda Acredolo and Susan Goodwyn, received grant money from the National Institutes of Health to study the long-term effects of teaching babies to communicate with gestures. They appeared on "Oprah," which is where I first learned about communicating with babies who can't yet speak. Their published research is a fascinating read on their findings. They found that after twenty-four months, the babies who were taught to gesture for what they wanted had vocabularies of twenty-eight-month-old babies and used longer sentences. The trend continued. When these same children were thirty-six months old, they spoke like forty-seven-month olds. Their continued research found that these children had better cognitive and language skills even when they were eight years old. They spoke better and had a better understanding of grammar and syntax. Additionally, the group that signed had IQ scores that averaged twelve points higher than those of children who did not. What lacked in their early book was a how-to guide for parents.

In addition Garcia and Acredolo and Goodwyn, there have been others who have researched and written about signing with babies. Dr. Marilyn Daniels' research shows that signing children have better recognition of letters and sounds. They are better spellers and have larger vocabularies. These same children are better readers and have more advanced communication skills. In her book *Dancing with Words*, she advocates incorporating ASL learning into the everyday school curriculum to improve reading literacy. Still other researchers continue to produce findings on signing and language learning. It is wonderful to see the broadening extent of the research, which is beginning to look at literacy in older children who sign.

Other books on signing with babies are listed in Appendix C.

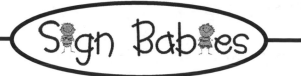

Appendix C

Resources

Sign Language Flash Cards for Babies and Children
Sign Language Flash Cards

Sign Babies ASL Flash Cards can be purchased at stores across the country or online at www.signbabies.com or call 1-800-456-0471.

Sign Babies ASL Flash Cards Set 1: First Words. Covers the twenty-five basic words babies and parents need most.

Sign Babies ASL Flash Cards Set 2: Around the House. Covers twenty-five signs for things around the house such as food, toys, and clothes.

Sign Babies ASL Flash Cards Set 3: Animals. Covers twenty-five signs for barnyard animals, zoo animals, and wild animals.

Sign Babies ASL Flash Cards Set 4: Family Life. Covers twenty-five signs for family members, manners, and emotions.

Learning Hands ASL Flash Cards: Food Fun. Covers twenty-five signs for food and drinks.

Learning Hands ASL Flash Cards: Let's Go! Covers twenty-five action signs such as swim, climb, sing, dance, and run.

Books for Children
Sign language books

Animal Signs by Debbie Slier. Pictures of animals and their signs.

Word Signs by Debbie Slier. Picture of words your baby wants to sign.

Baby's First Signs by Kim Votry and Curt Waller. Illustrated book of signs babies needs.

More Baby's First Signs by Kim Votry and Curt Waller. Illustrated book of signs babies needs.

A Book of Colors by Kim Votry and Curt Waller. Illustrated book of colors.

Out for a Walk by Kim Votry and Curt Waller. Illustrated book of things you find in your neighborhood.

General

Goodnight Moon by Margaret Wise Brown. A short poem of goodnight wishes from a young rabbit preparing for bed. He says goodnight to every object in sight.

Peeka-WHO? By Nina Laden. This simple, rhyming board book has alternating two-page spreads. "Peek a" is repeated, opposite an illustrated page with a die-cut hole, behind which lurks a cow (MOO!), zoo animals (ZOO!), a mirror (YOU!) and several other images.

Show Me! by Tom Tracy. A wonderful book about a mother dressing her baby and touching the baby's nose, cheeks, tummy and so forth.

My First Body Board Book by DK Publishing. Full-color photos of babies and body parts. This is a wonderful way to introduce the names of the body parts.

My First Word Book by DK Publishing. Full-color photos of words for the things your baby sees every day.

Pat the Bunny by Dorothy Kunhardt. The very first touch-and-feel book. It has been around since 1940 and is a classic.

Let's Play by Leo Lionni. Two mice ask each other, What shall we do today? They then discuss many possibilities of things that they can do such as read a book, pick flowers, go swimming, and play ball.

Food

Very Hungry Caterpillar by Eric Carle. The caterpillar emerges from his egg very hungry and proceeds to eat through everything he sees until he gets a stomach ache. He then builds a cocoon and waits to become a butterfly. Some of the foods are a bit obscure for baby signers–like pickle–but the book is so fun it is hard to resist.

Lunch by Denise Fleming. A very hungry mouse nibbles and crunches his way through a vegetarian feast, while your child is introduced to the individual foods and their respective colors.

Today Is Monday by Eric Carle. Each animal has a different thing to eat for a specific day of the week. At the end children are invited to come eat them all.

Animals

Moo, Baa La La La! by Sandra Boynton. A funny, rhyming romp through farm and neighborhood animals. This is one of the favorites at our house and can be quoted by everyone in unison.

Brown Bear, Brown Bear by Eric Carle. A very simple rhyme introduces baby to several animals and their colors. A wonderful book to sign.

Polar Bear, Polar Bear by Eric Carle. A wilder version of the simple rhyme in *Brown Bear, Brown Bear*. Even though the animals are not average ones your baby sees, the book is still fun to read. Use ANIMAL or a generic sign like BIRD when you don't know the sign for something such as peacock.

Good Night, Gorilla by Peggy Rathmann. This book has very simple text and wonderful illustrations about a gorilla who lets a whole zoo of animals loose. They end up in the zookeeper's bed. Don't be thrown by the armadillo and the hyena. Just sign ANIMAL.

Barnyard Dance! by Sandra Boynton. This book reads like a fun square dance call-out while it introduces barnyard animals.

Touch and Feel: Baby Animals by DK Publishing.

Touch and Feel: Farm by DK Publishing.

Touch and Feel: Wild Animals by DK Publishing.

Touch and Feel: Pets by DK Publishing.

DK Publishing excels at touch-and-feel books, and these are the best books for learning animals

Does a Kangaroo Have a Mother? by Eric Carle. This book teaches the names of several animals and the names of their babies.

There Was an Old Lady Who Swallowed a Fly by Simms Taback. This Caldecott Honor book is so wild that the craziness will make you laugh out loud. The cut outs let you see what the lady swallowed and the moral (never swallow a horse) will make you laugh. This book is for children two years and older.

Morning time

Hey! Wake Up by Sandra Boynton. This hilarious book introduces morning activities such as yawning, stretching, breakfast, getting dressed, and playtime.

Bedtime

The Going to Bed Book by Sandra Boynton. Our family's favorite bedtime book. An ark full of animals watches the sun go down and then prepares for bed. They take a bath, find pajamas, brush their teeth, do exercises up on deck, and finally say good night.

Pajama Time by Sandra Boynton. This book explores various sleep outfits that the animals put on before joining a pajama party. Everyone finally settles down, the lights are turned out, and wishes are shared for a hushed good night

Good Night, Gorilla by Peggy Rathmann. This book has very simple text and wonderful illustrations about a gorilla who lets a whole zoo of animals loose. They end up in the zookeeper's bed. Don't be thrown by the armadillo and the hyena. Just sign ANIMAL.

10 Minutes to Bedtime by Peggy Rathmann. Dad counts down the last ten minutes until his son has to go to bed. An entire community of hamsters joins a boy and his own pet hamster in getting ready for bed. Lots of action for you and your child to discuss. This book is better for children who are 2 years or older.

Clifford's Bedtime by Norman Bridwell. In this board book Clifford needs his blanket and favorite toys, a drink of water, and a good-night kiss. For children who love Clifford, this is a wonderful way to wind down.

Emotions/ behavior

Curious George Are You Curious? by H. A. Rey. This book illustrates a variety of emotions and states of being, including happy, proud, dizzy, naughty, silly, and curious.

Baby Faces by DK Publishing. This book captures the expressions and moods of babies throughout their busy days.

It's Neat to Eat at the Table by Lindy Bartell. One of the stories about Perry and Penny Pig and how they learn to have good manners.

Hands Are Not for Hitting by Martine Agassi. Teaches alternatives to hitting and ways of coping with and resolving strong feelings such as anger, jealousy, and fear.

I Love Hugs by Lara Jones. This book discusses different types of hugs like bear hugs today and make-it-better hugs.

Excuse Me! by Karen Katz. Introduces the magic words "Excuse me" and "I'm sorry" needed for situations from burping to breaking a sibling's toy. Your baby will have fun lifting the flaps to discover the right words to say.

Counting Kisses by Karen Katz. A fussy baby receives a different number of kisses from each member of the family—mom, dad, grandma, big sister, and even the dog and cat—that help her fall asleep.

Hug by Jez Alborough. A baby chimpanzee watches other animals get hugs. Through his expressions, we see several emotions as he searches for his own mother and his hug.

Kiss Kiss by Margaret Wild. Baby Hippo forgets to kiss his mama goodbye before he goes off to play. As he walks through the jungle, he sees other animal babies kissing their mothers, so he returns home and makes amends. A great book about separation and love.

Today I Feel Silly and Other Moods That Make My Day by Jamie Lee Curtis. A little girl tells about all her moods and shows how her face looks when she feels a certain way.

Colors/Descriptors/Numbers

Pajama Time by Sandra Boynton. This book explores various sleep outfits that the animals put on before joining a pajama party. Everyone finally settles down, the lights are turned out, and wishes are shared for a hushed good night

Brown Bear, Brown Bear by Eric Carle. A very simple rhyme introduces baby to several animals and their colors. A wonderful book to sign.

Lunch by Denise Fleming. A very hungry mouse nibbles and crunches his way through a vegetarian feast, while your child is introduced to the individual foods and their respective colors.

Counting Kisses by Karen Katz. A fussy baby receives a different number of kisses from each member of the family—mom, dad, grandma, big sister, and even the dog and cat—that help her fall asleep.

Blue Hat, Green Hat by Sandra Boynton. Animals introduce the basic colors and familiar items of clothing with a great touch of humor.

Oh My Oh My Oh Dinosaurs! by Sandra Boynton. This book teaches descriptor words and their opposites. Dinosaurs are tall and short, red and blue, and so forth.

What Makes a Rainbow? by Betty Ann Schwartz. A rainbow of ribbons magically appear when you open the pages of this innovative book. Teaches animals and colors.

Just for fun!

Belly Button Book by Sandra Boynton. This is a totally fun book that features a beachful of bare-bellied hippos—including one tiny baby who can only say "Bee Bo"—that love to show off their belly buttons.

Baby Faces by DK Publishing. This book capture the expressions and moods of babies throughout their busy days.

Peeka-WHO? by Nina Laden. This simple, rhyming board book has alternating two-page spreads. "Peek a" is repeated, opposite an illustrated page with a die-cut hole, behind which lurks a cow (MOO!), zoo animals (ZOO!), a mirror (YOU!) and several other images.

Books for Adults

Dictionary

Teach Your Tot to Sign by Stacy Thompson.

Other baby sign language books

Sign with Your BABY by Joseph Garcia. The man who started it all. Garcia's book was the first book to recommend using American Sign Language to communicate with hearing babies.

Baby Talk by Monica Beyer. Beyer's book is simple and easy to read with a basic dictionary. The illustrations are colorful and easy-to-understand

Sign, Sing, and Play!: Fun Signing Activities for You and Your Baby by Monta Z. Bryant.

IMPORTANT: *Baby Signs: How to Talk with Your Baby Before Your Baby Can Talk* by Linda Acredolo and Susan Goodwyn discusses much of the great research done by these wonderful women. However, some of the signs used in Baby Signs are *not* ASL signs. Hence, I recommend that you read this book for the uplifting stories and research information, but do not rely on the signs in the book if using only ASL signs is important to you.

Literacy and signing

Dancing with Words by Marilyn Daniels (2001). Westport, Connecticut: Bergin and Garvey.

Early childhood development

Caring for Your Baby and Young Child, Revised Edition: Birth to Age 5 by American Academy of Pediatrics.

Your Baby and Child: From Birth to Age Five by Penelope Leach.

The Baby Book: Everything You Need to Know About Your Baby from Birth to Age Two by William Sears, Martha Sears, Robert Sears, and James Sears.

What's Going on in There? How the Brain and Mind Develop in the First Five Years of Life by Lise Eliot.

Music

Pick Me Up! Activity Guide and Music CD. Contains twenty original songs that are entertaining for both parents and children and were specifically designed to sing and sign. Includes an activity guide with all the words and signs you need.

For the Kids. A wonderful CD of kid's songs sung by stars. A portion of the proceeds will help restore music education in the U.S. public school system through the VHI Save the Music Foundation. Songs that are great to sign include La La La La Lemon sung by the Barenaked Ladies, Hopity Song sung by Five for Fighting, and It's Alright to Cry sung by Darius Rucker.

Listen and Play: A great online resource for early learning songs comes from BBC Radio, which hosts Listen and Play, a twenty-eight audio resource for preschool children emphasizing the development of early literacy skills. Each program includes familiar songs, rhymes, stories, and sound discrimination games to develop children's phonological awareness and confidence with spoken language. The songs and games in this program can easily be adapted to using with your baby to enhance your experience in signing. See http://www.bbc.co.uk/schoolradio/earlylearning/listenandplay.shtml

Do-Rey-Me and You!

From the same people who created Kindermusik classes, Do-Rey-Me and You! CDs introduce various styles of music and have some wonderful songs to sign. Each CD comes with a book or an educational toy. For more on how to purchase the CDs, go to www.drmy.com.

10 in the Bed. A wonderful collection of songs that you can sign include "Ten in the Bed," "Five Little Ducks," "Old MacDonald," and "Mary Had a Little Lamb."

Mary Bridget's Surprise. Full of fun songs such as "Five Little Monkeys," "Home on the Range," "Sing Your Way Home," and "Monkey See, Monkey Do."

Mister Sun. Sunny songs that will make you both smile including "Sunshine on My Shoulders" and "You Are the Sunshine of My Life."

Critter Giggles. One of our favorites; includes "Place in the Choir," "Whadaliacha," and "The Green Grass Grew All Around." The joke book that accompanies the CD is too old for your child now, but when she is five, she will love them.

Tub Tunes. By far, the best collection of songs for the bath. It includes "Yellow Submarine," "Rub-a-Dub-Dub," and many other splashy favorites.

Head, Shoulders, Knees, and Toes. Includes "Head, Shoulders, Knees, and Toes," "If You're Happy and You Know It," and "I'm a Little Teapot," along with some other great songs such as "Locomotion" and "Them Bones."

Raffi

This is the music you hear in Gymboree. Some parents are annoyed by the guitar-playing Canadian, but kids love him and the songs are less annoying than many other musicians.

Singable Songs for the Very Young: Great with a Peanut-Butter Sandwich by Raffi. The CD includes several songs that are fun to sign, including "Brush Your Teeth," "Five Little Frogs," "Spider on the Floor," "Baa Baa Black Sheep," "Going to the Zoo," and "The Sharing Song."

Additionally, check out the Raffi books that go along with some classic songs, including *Spider on the Floor (Raffi Songs to Read)* by Raffi and True Kelley; *If You're Happy and You Know It (Raffi Songs to Read)* by Raffi and Cyd Moore; and *Five Little Ducks (Raffi Songs to Read)* by Raffi.

Puntumayo

Sing Along with Puntumayo. Features a star-studded cast of artists singing folk, blues, bluegrass, swing, and reggae that you can sign and sing, including a great jazzy version of "Old MacDonald" as well as a folk version of "You Are My Sunshine."

Folk Playground. A delightful collection of folk songs that introduces your baby to folk music. Even though you probably won't sign any songs on this CD, it is a wonderful CD to listen and dance to.

DVDs

The American Academy of Pediatrics suggests that children not be exposed to television before they are two years old. Their concern is that parents are using television as a babysitter for their children and that parents are lacking the direct interaction with their children. There is also some suggestion that extended television watching by children may change the way the brain is wired.

Having said that, there are several very good programs directed at teaching children American Sign Language signs. You are still your child's best teacher and your child will learn signs faster by interacting with you. However, you can supplement your child's learning experience by watching these videos with your child and interacting with them. By interacting with the videos, your child can see that you make the same signs that other children and parents are using. Seeing other children sign might help your child understand the signing process and get interested in learning more signs. Just use videos with caution and don't use them to babysit your child.

Signing time

Baby Signing Time. Created specifically to teach signing to the very young, *Baby Signing Time* combines songs, animation, and signing babies age two and under to make signing easy and fun.

Signing Time, Volumes 1–13. *Signing Time* works for both a young audience and for older siblings so if you have mixed ages, get these CDs instead of *Baby Signing Time*. Alex and Leah teach kids how to sign with the help of Rachel, beautiful music and animations. The CDs include great shots of other kids of all ages and abilities signing. You might also be able to catch *Signing Time* on your local PBS station.

Sign-A-Lot

Sign-A-Lot is a DVD series developed for hearing children ages two to eight, where American Sign Language vocabulary is woven into the storyline through an exciting, entertaining world of animated characters, magical lands and playful child performers. Through interactive signing games, your child will have fun signing along with the See Me Sign Kids as they travel to the magical land of Sign-A-Lot, where everything is "hands on." *Sign-A-Lot* inspires children to be participatory viewers, so get your imagination and hands ready to sign a lot!

Important Websites
Baby sign language websites

Sign Babies website: www.signbabies.com. Our website. It contains more information, stories, pictures, videos, podcasts, and more to help you with your signing experience.

Babies and Moms Radio: www.babiesandmomsradio.com. The website for the radio show that I host. We talk about signing with babies each week. You can check out podcasts or listen to us on iTunes. You can also see great videos of kids signing.

Sign2Me website: www.sign2me.com. A great place to find a class in your area.

Signing Baby: www.signingbaby.com. Created by a mom who signed with her kids, Signing Baby has great information for parents.

ASL dictionaries

American Sign Language Browser from Michigan State University: commtechlab.msu.edu/sites/aslweb/browser.htm. A great way to see signs you want to learn.

ASL University: www.lifeprint.com. Dr. Vicars' online courses also has a pretty good dictionary you can check for signs.

Online ASL courses

ASL University: www.lifeprint.com. Dr. Vicars' online course on ASL is not the prettiest, but he has good content and great clips, and it is free unless you need credits.

Signing Online Interactive Web-based Instruction: www.signingonline.com. An online course that costs a nominal fee, but is very good. Students who tested it like this course better and would be willing to pay for it.

Deaf Culture

Deaf Culture Online: www.deaf-culture-online.com/deafculture.html. A great resource for learning more about deaf culture.

Other Resources on Development
ASHA website

The American Speech-Language-Hearing Association (ASHA) has a wealth of information for parents on how speech and language develop. This is a great site to learn what your child should be doing at a specific age and what to look for if you suspect that your child is delayed. www.asha.org.

Zero to Three

This website is an amazing resource of information for parents on the first three years of your child's life. www.zerotothree.org

One of the best sections is called Brain Wonders www.zerotothree.org/brainwonders) and it explains what is going on inside your baby's brain during each developmental age group. There are two sections for each age group: *What's Going On* that alerts you to the latest information about brain development and *What You Can Do* that gives you strategies to support your baby's development.

Another wonderful section is called The Magic of Everyday Moments (www.zerotothree.org/magic); it explains how daily activities, such as feeding, bathing, and grocery shopping can be rich opportunities to encourage your child's development by building self-confidence, curiosity, social skills, self-control, and communication skills.

Born Learning

Born Learning (www.bornlearning.org/) helps you shape your child's world and understand that everyday life is a learning experience. Reading through this site helps you understand how to incorporate learning in to everything you do. The Ages and Stages series of PDF files on this site is an excellent review of where your child is at during every stage.

Parents as Teachers

Parents as Teachers (PAT) is a parent education and family support program serving families throughout pregnancy until their child enters kindergarten, usually age five (www.parentsasteachers.org/). In your local area, there may be a chapter of Parents as Teachers that provides services and education to help you learn more about being a parent. For example, in my local area, PAT sets up monthly home visits with new mothers to help support and educate them.

Healthy Start

U.S. Department of Education Healthy Start Brochures designed to help you understand your child's needs. www.ed.gov/parents/earlychild/ready/healthystart/index.html

Today's Mama

Today's Mama is a wonderful portal to great information for moms. Local information is included on classes and activities for both mothers and babies. www.todaysmama.com.

Research on Signing with Hearing Children

A longitudinal study funded by the National Institutes of Child Health and Human Development showed that babies who used symbolic gestures understood more words, had larger vocabularies, and engaged in more sophisticated play than nonsigning babies. Parents of the signing babies in the study noted decreased frustration, increased communication, and enriched parent-infant bonding. Signing babies also displayed an increased interest in books. Researchers revisited the families in the original study when the children were seven and eight years old. The children who signed as babies had a mean IQ of 114 compared to the nonsigning control group's mean IQ of 102.

Researchers have also found that hearing students in pre-kindergarten classes who receive instruction in both English and ASL score significantly higher on the Peabody Picture Vocabulary Test than hearing students in classes with no sign instruction. Specifically, the studies of Dr. Marilyn Daniels demonstrate that adding visual and kinesthetic elements to verbal communication helps enhance a preschool child's vocabulary, spelling, and reading skills.

Acredolo, L. P., Goodwyn, S. W., & Brown, Catherine. (2000). "Impact of Symbolic Gesturing on Early Language Development" *Journal of Nonverbal Behavior*, 24, 81–103.

Acredolo, L. P., and Goodwyn, S. W. (July 2000). "The Long-Term Impact of Symbolic Gesturing during Infancy on IQ at Age 8." Paper presented at the meetings of the International Society for Infant Studies, Brighton, UK.

Anthony, M. E. (2002). "The Role of American Sign Language and 'Conceptual Wholes' in Facilitating Language, Cognition, and Literacy." PhD dissertation, University of California, Berkeley.

Daniels, M. (October 1994). "The Effects of Sign Language on Hearing Children's Language Development." *Communication Education*, 43(4), 291.

Daniels, M. (1996). "Seeing Language: The Effect Over Time of Sign Language on Vocabulary Development in Early Childhood Education." *Child Study Journal*, 26, 193–208.

Daniels, M. (2001). *Dancing with Words: Signing for Hearing Children's Literacy*. Westport, Connecticut: Bergin and Garvey.

Feltzer, Laura. MBR Reading Program: How Signing Helps Hearing Children Learn to Read. Research Summary.

Felzer, L. (1998). "A Multisensory Reading Program That Really Works." *Teaching and Change*, 5, 169–183.

Goldstein, M. H., and West, M. J. (1999). "Consistent Responses of Human Mothers to Prelinguistic Infants: The Effect on Prelinguistic Repertoire Size," *Journal of Comparative Psychology*, 113, 52–58.

Grabmeier, J. (1999). "Infants Use Sign Language to Communicate at Ohio State School." Newswise Press. http://www.newswise.com/articles/view/?id=SIGNLANG.OSU.

Hafer, J. (1986). *Signing for Reading Success*. Washington, D.C.: Clerc Books, Gallaudet University Press.

Koehler, L., and Loyd, L. (September 1986). Using Fingerspelling/Manual Signs to Facilitate Reading and Spelling. Biennial Conference of the International Society for Augmentative and Alternative Communication. (4th, Cardiff, Wales).

Moore, Brie, Acredolo, Linda, and Goodwyn, Susan. (April 2001). Symbolic gesturing and joint attention: Partners in facilitating verbal development. Paper presented at the Biennial Meetings of the Society for Research in Child Development.

Wilson, R., Teague, J., and Teague, M. (1985). "The Use of Signing and Fingerspelling to Improve Spelling Performance with Hearing Children." *Reading Psychology*, 4, 267–273.

Research on Signing with Special Needs Children
Apraxia of speech

Gretz, Sharon. Using Sign Language with Children Who Have Apraxia of Speech: Available online at www.apraxia-kids.org/topics/sign.html.

Square, P. A. (1994). "Treatment Approaches for Developmental Apraxia of Speech." *Clinical Communications Disorders*, 4(3), 151–161.

Autism

Stephen M. Edelson, Ph.D., from the Center for the Study of Autism, Salem, Oregon writes:

"Many aberrant behaviors associated with autism and other developmental disabilities, such as aggression, tantrumming, self-injury, anxiety, and depression, are often attributed to an inability to communicate to others. Signed Speech may, at the very least, allow the person to communicate using signs and may stimulate verbal language skills. When teaching a person to use sign language, another possible benefit may be the facilitation of their attentiveness to social gestures of others as well as of themselves."

Dr. Edelson's article is available online at www.autism.org/sign.html.

Down syndrome

Donovan, Claire. (1998). "Teaching Sign Language." *Disability Solutions*, 2(5).

Gibbs, E. D., Springer, A. S., Cooley, S. C. & Aloisio, S. (November 1991). Early Use of Total Communication: Patterns across Eleven Children with Down Syndrome. Paper presented at the meeting of the International Early Childhood Conference on Children with Special Needs, St. Louis, MO.

Hopmann, Marita R. (1993). "The Use of Signs by Children with Down Syndrome." *Down Syndrome Today*, 2(2), 22–23. Available online at www.csdsa.org/artsigns.htm.

Miller J. F., Sedey, A., Miolo, G., Rosin, M., & Murray-Branch, J. (August 1992). Vocabulary Acquisition in Young Children with Down

Syndrome: Speech and Sign. Paper presented at the 9th World Congress of the International Association for the Scientific Study of Mental Deficiency (Queensland, Australia).

Watson, Claire. (Winter 1996). "Total Communication Options for Children with Down Syndrome in the Context of Hanen Programs for Parents." *Wig Wag.* Available online at www.altonweb.com/cs/downsyndrome/watson.html.

Reading disabilities

Blackburn, D., Vonvillian, J., & Ashby, R. (January 1984). "Manual Communication as an Alternative Mode of Language Instruction for Children with Severe Reading Disabilities." *Language, Speech and Hearing Services in Schools*, 15, 22–31.

Carney, J., Cioffi, G., & Raymond, W. (Spring 1985). "Using Sign Language for Teaching Sight Words." *Teaching Exceptional Children*, 214–217.

Sensenig, L., Topf, B., & Mazeika, E. (June 1989). "Sign Language Facilitation of Reading with Students Classified as Trainable Mentally Handicapped." *Education and Training of the Mentally Retarded*, 121–125.

Vernon, M., Coley, J., Hafer, J., & Dubois, J. (April 1980). "Using Sign Language to Remediate Severe Reading Problems." *Journal of Learning Disabilities*, 13, 215–218.

Children in hospital settings

Hall, S.S. & Weatherly, K.S. (1989). "Using Sign Language with Tracheotomized Infants and Children." *Pediatric Nurse*, 15(4): 362–367. Available online at www.ncbi.nlm.nih.gov.

Index